Reclaiming
Your Body

Also by Suzanne Scurlock-Durana

Full Body Presence:
Learning to Listen to Your Body's Wisdom

Reclaiming Your Body

Healing from Trauma and
Awakening to Your Body's Wisdom

SUZANNE SCURLOCK-DURANA

New World Library
Novato, California

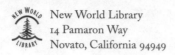

New World Library
14 Pamaron Way
Novato, California 94949

Text design by Tona Pearce Myers

Library of Congress Cataloging-in-Publication Data
Names: Scurlock-Durana, Suzanne, [date]– author.
Title: Reclaiming your body : healing from trauma and awakening to your body's
   wisdom / Suzanne Scurlock-Durana.
Description: Novato, California : New World Library, [2017] | Includes
   bibliographical references and index.
Identifiers: LCCN 2017000435 (print) | LCCN 2017006593 (ebook) | ISBN
   9781608684687 (paperback) | ISBN 9781608684694 (Ebook)
Subjects: LCSH: Craniosacral therapy. | Mind and body. | BISAC: BODY, MIND
   & SPIRIT / Healing / General. | SELF-HELP / Personal Growth / General. |
   PSYCHOLOGY / Psychopathology / Post-Traumatic Stress Disorder (PTSD). |
   HEALTH & FITNESS / Alternative Therapies.
Classification: LCC RZ399.C73 S382 2017 (print) | LCC RZ399.C73 (ebook) | DDC
   615.8/528—dc23
LC record available at https://lccn.loc.gov/2017000435

First printing, June 2017
ISBN 978-1-60868-468-7
Ebook ISBN 978-1-60868-469-4
Printed in Canada on 100% postconsumer-waste recycled paper

New World Library is proud to be a Gold Certified Environmentally Responsible Publisher. Publisher certification awarded by Green Press Initiative. www.greenpressinitiative.org

10   9   8   7   6   5   4   3   2

To my mom, Mary Jane,
for her indomitable spirit and her love of life

Contents

Preface

The information in this book was born over three decades ago out of my own healing and my exploration into what was needed to facilitate that healing. In that time I have practiced and taught CranioSacral Therapy (CST), which is a gentle hands-on technique, originally practiced only by osteopaths but now taught and practiced by a wide range of healthcare providers. It utilizes light touch and engages the body's wisdom and healing potential through a series of physical and emotional releases. During this therapy, you mobilize the bones and membranes of the brain and spinal cord. My mentor was Dr. John Upledger, and I have taught for the Upledger Institute since 1986. I tell the story of how I discovered and trained in this work in chapter 11.

CST healed *my* chronic pain and sent me on a mission to uncover more about how we can truly become friends again with our own body. In my healing process all those years ago, I discovered that my cells hold wisdom that is just waiting to be listened to. And listen I have — more and more closely to all parts of myself. By using my body's wisdom — listening to and being present in my heart, my gut, my pelvis, and my bones for healing and guidance — I developed the program I call "Healing from the Core" (HFC) to share this internal body wisdom and experience with others.

The stories in this book are all real examples of cellular intelligence, awakened by my HFC work alone or combined with CST. I am unabashedly biased in this realm. My hope is that, once you are shown how revolutionary this is, and you give it a real chance, you will agree. There is no doubt in my mind or body as to its validity and efficacy.

However, our culture as a whole does not always see what is so obvious to me. All the recent breakthroughs in brain research and trauma (which I describe later) were thought to be heresy as little as ten to twenty years ago. When I teach this work in a new professional group, I often assume people know and understand about their body's wisdom. How could you miss it? It is so simple and obvious to me.

And yet, again and again, I am shocked to witness exactly the opposite. The good news is that people these days now understand the central concepts. They understand why they might want to be grounded and centered and that yoga and meditation bring these concepts to life. *Presence* is a huge buzzword in the coaching and psychotherapy world, and our awareness of being in the present moment has been growing ever since Ram Dass pointed it out to us decades ago. My own healing work and the explorations in this book build on these concepts.

Still, many people have never actually had the *experience*, and this work is all about the experience — the direct experience of full-body presence and body wisdom — what it feels like, tastes like, smells like, and looks like. Beyond our five senses, it is also the ineffable *experience* of simply being alive, which encompasses our body, mind, and spirit. Many people don't even realize what they are missing. Yet without being present in our body, our experience just is not the same. It is severely limited. It's like a building without a solid foundation. My hope is that this book helps you build that foundation.

1 The Answers Lie Within
The Journey Begins

I have been and still am a seeker, but I have ceased to question stars and books; I have begun to listen to the teaching my blood whispers to me.

— HERMANN HESSE

Compared to what we ought to be, we are only half awake. Our fires are damped, our drafts are checked. We are making use of only a small part of our possible mental and physical resources.

— WILLIAM JAMES

The body has its own language that is older and more primal than most of us realize. Our bodies speak to us with sensations, images, emotions, and an inner knowing that is beyond words. Have you ever had a niggling doubt that nags you for days, a vague pain in your leg that won't go away, or a heaviness in your heart that could mean either "I need to call my mother" or "I should call my doctor"? This book will help you understand what these sensations mean and how to respond to them.

Common idioms, the little everyday phrases that people use, often capture glimpses of this body wisdom. For instance, "my

1

heart goes out to you" is obviously not meant literally. It is a figure of speech that means "I am feeling empathy for you and am reaching out to connect." But when you hear or read those words, how do they make you *feel*? When I read "my heart goes out to you," I feel a rush of warmth in my chest, and I soften. My chest expands as I contemplate my heart energetically encompassing someone in need.

Most of us are conditioned at a very young age to turn off this inner guidance system of sensation, imagery, and inner knowing. Our priceless body wisdom is getting lost as our culture speeds up and becomes more technology driven. Compounding this issue is the fact that life's traumas also cut us off from our body's wisdom.

As a result, we may flounder when making decisions, we may remain in less-than-ideal or unsafe situations, and we may end up living a life that truly isn't ours — while the whole time our body is madly signaling us with the answers and solutions we seek.

Now is the time to start listening! This book is about reclaiming this life-giving system that lies within each of us, patiently waiting to be heard.

The Beginnings of My Disconnection

When I was a young child, I felt connected to my body. I ran through the grass, climbed trees, built forts, and played outside every day and into the evenings. My heart felt as big as the sky, and life touched me deeply.

One warm autumn day, when I was almost four, a dog wandered into our front yard, and I felt an immediate bond with this gentle, golden-haired creature. It was as though we had known each other forever. I hugged him as we rolled in the grass and snuggled together for hours. I was certain this wonderful four-legged being was going to be my lifelong friend.

When I took him into the house to share my excitement, my

parents informed me that I could not keep him — the dog must surely belong to someone else, and we had to find his owner.

I was shocked! I cried so hard I could barely breathe. Couldn't they see how deeply connected we were? How could they separate me from my newly discovered old friend? I still remember the warmth in his eyes and the deep connection we shared at a heart level.

This experience sent the message that heart connections didn't matter. My natural capacity for joy and exuberance was diminished that day.

As the eldest of my family's three children, I was shuttled off to kindergarten at age four before I was emotionally ready. On my first day in that huge, dark old building, my mom reassured me that if I didn't like it, she would be waiting outside to take me home.

Ten minutes into class, as I looked at the dour, unsmiling face of Mrs. Hoyberger, I knew deep inside that I did not belong there. This world felt closed in, dry, and regimented. I quietly slipped into the cloakroom and then out the classroom door. Down the hall I ran, looking for my mom. The outside door was so heavy it took all my strength to open it, but I was determined.

Once outside, I was devastated to discover that my mom had left without me. Just then, Mrs. Hoyberger grabbed me from behind and sternly ushered me back to the classroom, from which there was no further escape.

On that day, I learned to rein in my tears and my sense of being overwhelmed in order to fit in. As I grew, I began to shut down other parts of myself to create an acceptable and pleasing persona for my family and teachers.

My fear of new endeavors became a pattern that stayed with me for decades. In college, I realized that once I started a project, I was fine. But during the weeks prior to starting, I felt an anxiety that could mentally paralyze me.

Another message I internalized was that no one would actually be there to catch me if I fell — so I could truly depend *only* on myself. This belief made me stronger and more self-reliant, but it became harder to let other people in because I regarded my vulnerability as a liability — something to hold at arm's length.

I was very observant and smart. I learned that when I placed my needs last and took care of everyone else first, I gained approval and love. I learned to value my intelligent, reasoning mind more than the feelings and sensations of my body.

My mother was the classic good wife of the 1950s, one who was subservient to her husband. My father, a Baptist minister, was a kind man and a deep thinker, an excellent speaker, and much loved by his congregation.

I modeled myself after my father, the parent who held all the power. I did not want to be like my mother. In the process, I didn't realize I was moving away from my authentic self, bit by bit.

At the age of six, I remember getting the tip of my right pinkie finger crushed by the chain on our backyard swing set. Screaming at the top of my lungs, I ran into the house, blood streaming from what remained of the end of my finger.

My father quickly cleaned and dressed the wound, gently and carefully wrapping it in gauze and taping it. Then he quietly let me know that I needed to stop crying — just like that!

I *so* aspired to be the person my dad wanted me to be. My finger hurt like hell, but I knew that if I wanted to please him, I needed to put a lid on my pain and stop crying. So I did.

Given all this, I'm not surprised to look back now and see that, by the time I was a teenager, I lived behind invisible walls, firmly shielded from whatever I thought could possibly hurt me.

I rarely cried, only doing so when I was alone. I saw myself as the "Rock of Gibraltar," a place of safety and strength for everyone who needed me. People loved me for my responsible caregiving, while within I felt numb and confused. The tenderness in my own heart did not get seen, much less touched. I was constantly trying to please everyone.

Mine is not an uncommon story. My traumas were not large, relatively speaking. Some might not consider them traumas at all. I certainly have been witness to friends and clients in my therapeutic practice and classes who have experienced *far* worse.

Yet trauma is a subjective experience. We should not judge our own traumas as being large or small by comparing them with anyone else's experience — not even doctors can know the personal impact of an individual's experiences and how they may be stored in their system.

As I travel and teach internationally, I ask my students if they consider their empathy and sensitivity to life to be an *asset*. Very few hands go up. Most of us consider our empathic abilities a *liability*, not an asset. Few realize that this internal capacity to feel life is what makes us fully human and allows us to function to our full potential. What I mean by healthy empathy is the capacity to sense our body, our emotions, and to walk in someone else's shoes without taking on their issues as our own.

Ironically, despite caring about others and our empathetic responses, when we create excessive protective barriers between the world and ourselves, we unknowingly undermine ourselves. We don't realize that these barriers may sometimes shield us from life's pain, but they also cut us off from the juiciness of life, from our creativity and joy, and from the knowing that helps us take care of ourselves.

One hot, humid summer night when I was seventeen, I got a pivotal wake-up call that fundamentally changed the direction of my life. That evening was a typical Virginia summer night. The air felt thick and heavy. I was at a neighborhood pool party. My friend John asked if we could go somewhere and talk. I thought the request was a bit odd, but I figured he needed some sisterly advice.

John was a longtime friend, a sweet teddy bear of a guy. Unbeknownst to me, he was spinning out of control in that moment and coming down from a long stretch on amphetamines. I was clueless about the underground drug culture that was widespread around me.

We sat in the front seat of his car in the parking lot outside the pool and were having a normal teenage conversation, just "hanging out." As we talked, I began to feel a strange but distinct uneasiness in my gut. This was not in response to the tone of his voice or the topic of conversation, yet the uneasiness continued for well over half an hour.

My *thoughts* were telling me it was unreasonable to feel uncomfortable with my friend, so I ignored my *gut feelings*. After all, he was like an older brother to me, and I dismissed my discomfort as foolish and didn't say anything about it.

Then, I turned away from him for a moment to look out the window, and the next thing I knew his hands were around my throat. He was strangling me. He was so strong I quickly and completely passed out.

When I regained consciousness, I was trembling all over. My head was pressed against the car door. John was plastered to the other side of the front seat, behind the steering wheel, obviously shocked and horrified at what he had done. He was apologizing profusely. I, too, was in serious shock.

Every cell in my body screamed at me to get out of the car *now*. This time, I listened. My primal survival instinct overruled my sweet seventeen-year-old politeness. As the strength in the lower half of my body surged back, I managed to open the door, and I crawled, shaking like a leaf, across the parking lot to my boyfriend's car, where help was waiting.

My heart felt shattered. Afterward, I soon learned why my friend had been so violent that night; he had been on drugs and was basically melting down inside. But my mental, left-brained knowing could not fix the damage. It took years of bodywork and emotional healing to melt the internal scars of fear and betrayal from that event.

In the moment, had I recognized and appreciated my gut intelligence and honored the message it was giving me, I could have avoided this life-changing trauma.

By saying this, I am not implying that what happened was my fault! This is a common response among trauma survivors, as I know from my decades of study and work with this population. Survivors may blame themselves, especially when the perpetrator is someone they know. In the immediate aftermath of my encounter, I did the same thing, wondering what it was *about me* that had caused this to happen.

Yet the blame was not mine, and I want to be clear that victims are not to blame for their traumas. Life happens, and even in the best of situations, we are never fully in control.

On the other hand, I also learned something valuable that forms the core of what I want to share with you in this book. This lesson can help you make the best decisions possible, regardless of external conditions and circumstances.

As I healed emotionally and physically from my traumatic experience, I became fascinated with the realization that *my gut had known that something was off about sitting in that car with my friend!*

Afterward, I promised myself that I would never second-guess my gut knowing again, even if the reasons for that knowing were not readily apparent on any other level.

That experience opened my eyes, and I realized that I had failed to listen to my own alarm system. My learned habits, automatic responses, and limiting beliefs had kept me from listening to and acting on my body's wisdom.

This life-threatening trauma jolted me awake and brought me to my process of self-healing. The journey home to the wisdom of my body is my life's work, and it is this process I share with you in this book. Not only did it enable me to heal fully, but it also has guided me in ways that helped me avoid other potentially traumatizing situations.

I hope that as more people awaken to the wisdom that lies within, fewer will experience the kind of trauma I did.

The Most Important Relationship in Your Life

Your relationships with other people throughout your lifetime — with your parents, spouses, children, friends, and teachers — will shift as time passes and situations change. As long as you are alive, however, your body is always with you.

It is so beneficial to have a strong, deep, intimate relationship with your own unique physical self.

Your body is designed to guide you, keep you safe, and bring you full vitality and pleasure. It is the vehicle through which you create and manifest your thoughts and dreams into reality.

In this book, you will discover how establishing and nurturing a healthy relationship with your body will allow you to reclaim lost parts of yourself, tap into your body's wisdom, and better navigate your life.

Let's begin by exploring your current relationship with your body, first by discovering what I call your "Body IQ," or "BQ" for short. This simple baseline assessment reveals how comfortable you are in your own skin. While my main goal is to help you develop a better relationship with your body, *awareness of where you stand now is the first step.*

Please engage your curiosity and suspend your judgment as you answer the nine questions in the "BQ: Body Intelligence Quiz."

BQ: Body Intelligence Quiz

Is your current relationship with your body friendly, or does it feel uneasy or unsettled? Take this nine-question quiz to find out. Don't overthink your answers. Just circle the number that best expresses your quick "first hit" response.

1. When you think about your body...
    Is your first impulse to feel appreciation for it?
    Or do you judge yourself and mostly notice things you want to change?

    Appreciation ←—————————→ **Judgment**
    1   2   3   4   5

2. When you engage in a typical daily activity...
    Are you more likely to trust that you know what you are doing?
    Or do you feel fearful about the outcome?

    Trust ←—————————→ **Fear**
    1   2   3   4   5

3. When a stressful situation arises...
    Do you calmly and clearly problem-solve the issue, the way you might talk it over with a friend?
    Or are you more likely to get confused and anxious?

    Calm ←—————————→ **Anxious**
    1   2   3   4   5

Continued on next page

4. When your body's natural needs and urges arise for sleep, food, fluids, sex, and elimination...
   Do you feel at peace with those needs?
   Or are you at odds or in conflict with your body?

   Peace ← ————————————→ Conflict

   1   2   3   4   5

5. When you are stepping into something new in your life...
   Do you feel supported by your body?
   Or do you feel it betrays you by putting the brakes on?

   Support ← ————————————→ Betrayal

   1   2   3   4   5

6. When your body has physical issues and/or you become ill...
   Do you have clarity and understanding about the nature of those issues?
   Or do you feel confused and unsure about their origins?

   Clarity ← ————————————→ Confusion

   1   2   3   4   5

7. When you slow down and turn your attention inward...
   Do you feel deeply connected to your body and its needs?
   Or do you feel detached, as though you are watching someone else?

   Connected ← ————————————→ Detached

   1   2   3   4   5

8. When someone tells you something about yourself...
   Do you trust your own inner reflections and what
   you know to be true?
   Or do you automatically accept what they have said
   because you do not know what *is* true for yourself?

   Trust Yourself ←——————→ **Believe Others**

1	2	3	4	5

9. When you are in action, thinking and doing in your
   world...
   Are you in easy partnership with your body?
   Or do you see your body as something you have to
   control — masterfully riding it until it does what you
   want?

   In Partnership ←——————→ **Controlling**

1	2	3	4	5

Add up your circled numbers for all nine questions. If
your score is low (under 18), you probably feel pretty
comfortable in your own skin under most circumstances.
If your score is between 18 and 28, your feelings of connection to your body are probably more variable. If your
score is on the high side (28 or more), your relationship
with your body may not be what you want it to be, but
rest assured *you are not alone*.

Whatever your BQ score, we all live in a culture where
disconnection from the sensations and signals of our bodies is
rampant. The latest research on trauma and healing — which is
spoken about so eloquently in *The Body Keeps Score* by Bessel van
der Kolk[1] and *In an Unspoken Voice* by Peter Levine[2] — shows that
the natural first response of the body to traumatic challenges in
life is to prepare to fight or flee.

If that is not possible, we tighten down, go into protection mode, and often numb out completely. Simply put, when we are helpless to stop a traumatic event, we shrink down inside or emotionally vacate the premises, freezing or dissociating, and we may even go into complete paralysis.

Once the initial trauma is over, these innate responses don't always pass. Instead, they may haunt us for years. The brilliant navigational system of our body may be deeply compromised.

This wonderful, innate system includes the following parts:

Our heart's capacity for inspiration, compassion, and joy
Our gut knowing
The powerful engine of our pelvis
The metabolizing capacities of our limbs (particularly
    our legs and feet)
The steadiness of our bones

These parts of ourselves are designed to work in partnership with one another — and with the triage areas of the brain. When unresolved trauma is lodged inside, blocking the way, the ability of this exquisite system to share its wisdom and strategies may no longer function properly.

No submarine could operate without its sonar, no driver without maps and signs. Yet most of us arrive at adulthood with many of our inner signal readers numbed out — or totally blocked.

Is It Safe or Dangerous? Pleasurable or Painful?

Dr. Stephen Porges, in his landmark work *The Polyvagal Theory*,[3] talks about how humans operate optimally when we feel safe and connected to the world around us. His polyvagal research and theory have brought to light how healthy vagus nerve function is what helps us feel happy and connected to life.

The vagus nerve regulates the entire "rest-and-digest" part of the nervous system — the parasympathetic branch — stimulating everything from the salivary glands in the mouth to the beating of the heart to full digestion and elimination — in other words, from one end of the system to the other.

When the sympathetic part of the nervous system, the "fight-or-flight" impulse, is operating, it suppresses the functioning of the parasympathetic branch and the vagus. From an evolutionary perspective, this helped us outrun the tiger. Our bodies shifted from digesting our lunch to working our legs so we wouldn't become lunch!

However, this means that in today's world most of us are not operating from healthy vagal functioning due to the daily stressors in our lives as well as to past unresolved trauma. This in turn inhibits our "rest-and-digest" system, as well as the social engagement system that gives us a deeper sense of connection in each moment, which we all need for a better quality of life.

When the body's core systems are not registering safety and nurturing connection, all our systems slow down and become depleted, leaving us in a constant state of hypervigilance, always on the lookout for the next threat.[4]

The bad news is that this epidemic of disconnection is everywhere. Look around and you'll see that many people are more connected to their technology or their "to-do" list than to their loved ones.

Check out the number of parents who are on their cell phones while they are out with their children. Notice the couples checking email in a restaurant rather than talking to each other. You may even feel overwhelmed yourself, rushing through life and yet missing the joy because of a busy schedule.

Today we spend more time worrying about the future or being haunted by the past than living in the present moment. Sadly, the more trauma you have experienced, the more disconnected you may feel. But even if you have not experienced serious trauma, life in our fast-paced culture can disconnect us.

The good news is that this is repairable in a number of ways. Neuroscience confirmed the concept of neuroplasticity in the 1990s. This means that, throughout life, our brain and nervous system can grow, heal, and remodel.

Reclaiming Your Navigational System

My work for the last three decades has been about reclaiming all of who we are to restore our natural balance and our innate healing potential. Peter Levine says it so clearly, "Trauma is a fact of life. It does not, however, have to be a life sentence."[5]

While your path home to yourself is unique, all paths include your body and the capacity to feel the sensations of being alive within your skin.

The journey of reclaiming these instinctual parts of who we are is an exciting exploration. In each of the upcoming chapters, you will discover a new skill that you can practice until it is mastered.

You will then be on *your* way to having a healthy relationship with your inner navigational system. You will have access to the vital, primal information your body provides.

Your inner radar will be up and running *and* fully functional.

Once most of your system is available to you again, you can easily navigate the rest of the way home as you go about living your life through openness and curiosity rather than from fear and anxiety.

Consider questions like these as you go about your day:

- What food would nourish me right now?
- Is this a healthy exchange I'm having, or do I need to speak up for myself or remove myself from this situation?
- What is my next step in this relationship?

When we're in tune with our body wisdom, these questions become simple, curiosity-stimulating avenues that lead us back to our body — our home, our refuge, our safe place — without a lot of charge or angst.[6]

You can begin to feel the exquisite joy of connecting to life: the beauty of a flower or a landscape, the love of a pet, or the connection you feel with a friend or your beloved.

2

The Five Body Myths

Blind Alleys That Throw Us Off Course

Don't let your mind bully your body.

— ASTRID ALAUDA

Having a good relationship with one's body is clearly important. Yet I know that somehow I lost touch with mine, and I know that I am not alone in this dilemma.

After several millennia, the Western world has left many of us partially or completely divorced from our body sensations and wisdom. Whatever the reason — whether we blame Descartes or trace this back to the fall of the ancient goddess traditions and the rise of patriarchy — the results are the same.

Many of our religions and spiritual traditions speak of being wary of the body, controlling the body, rising above the body, and most of all, putting the body in a subservient role to the mind. In numerous ways, we are taught the body is "less than" our thoughts and mental faculties.

In the thousands of interviews I have conducted and healing sessions I have facilitated over the last three decades, I have seen that this loss of good relationship with the body is pretty universal, and it can cause major mental, emotional, physical, and spiritual problems.

First and foremost, not feeling connected to our body leaves us very vulnerable. We get anxious even when there is actually nothing to fear. We unknowingly put ourselves in harm's way. We lose out on the opportunities for joy in each moment. If we are not connected to our body's wisdom, we miss inner signals that are vital for surviving and thriving in today's world.

All of us operate from a variety of body myths and either unconsciously or consciously believe them to be true. Body myths are often handed down to us through our family lineage. Below, I've identified five body myths based on my experiences, conversations with peers, and the stories shared in my trainings and private sessions across the last three decades. These may not all seem true for you at the same time; some may seem partially true; or some might have felt true at a particular time.

However, these are myths that you probably do not want to continue living from if you have a choice. The first step in this process is awareness. With awareness, we are given the possibility of choosing anew.

Body Myth 1: The Body Is Too Painful

Numerous students have said to me: "When I turn my attention inward, all I feel is pain, and I feel overwhelmed. I don't know how to deal with my pain, so I don't want to — I can't handle anything more. How can feeling this pain more than I already do possibly be helpful?"

If any of this sounds familiar, ask yourself these questions:

Do I view my inner pain as an insurmountable problem?
Do I feel only anxiety when I drop inside?
Do I feel like my pain is bigger than me?

Many people who have survived traumatic, overwhelming events may have this initial response when they drop their awareness to sensations within their own inner landscape. The pain is real. *That* part is definitely not a myth, though we may have been told it was. The myth comes in believing that the pain is *all that inhabits our insides.*

All I Am Is This Huge Ball of Pain...

Jennifer was newly separated from her husband of ten years when she came to one of my classes. She was an attractive, well-dressed woman whose sweetness shone through her face and eyes. The tension in her shoulders and back told me that she was also carrying an inner burden of pain.

As the class started and it was her turn to share, she began to cry. Through her tears, she told us that although she was firm in her decision to divorce her husband, every time she stopped to reflect on it, she became overwhelmed with a deep ache in her midsection. When I asked her more about the size and shape of the pain, she described it as a "watermelon-size ball of excruciating grief." It brought her to a flood of tears just describing it. I acknowledged her pain and how that huge, contracted ache in her midsection must be controlling her life.

To help her come out of feeling so overwhelmed, I asked her to notice how her backbone felt resting into her chair. She relaxed slightly as she allowed her awareness to expand to that area. I asked her to notice the weight of her ribs and spine as she rested back even more. Her flood of tears started to slow down as her pain lessened.

Next, I asked about the sensation of her sitting bones on the chair. As this awareness settled in, she spoke through her tears, "I am all alone without support now that I have struck out on my own. Even my family is upset with me for leaving my great provider of a husband."

I didn't know most of the facts regarding her current situation. However, I did know that she had come to my circle with two friends, who were sitting on either side of her. I asked her to allow her awareness to spread out to either side so that she could feel the supportive presence of her friends. As she explored this possibility, her tears slowed to a trickle.

Next, I suggested that she direct her attention to the sensation of her feet resting on the floor and, within the ease of this connection, to simply notice how supportive it felt. Gravity connects us to the earth, without any effort, in every moment of our lives. This resource is available to everyone, although few are conscious of it. This awareness seemed to shift something inside that turned the tide of her grief.

Finally, I asked her how that watermelon-size ball of grief in her midsection was doing. She got very quiet, and her mouth curled into a smile as she reported that it was about the size of an orange and that she was feeling much better. We had dispelled Body Myth 1, and she now had more of herself to compassionately hold her sadness and grief.

Body Myth 2: The Body Is Mysterious and Dangerous

I grew up with Body Myth 2. I was raised in a good Southern Baptist family with lots of wonderful singing, praising of God, and the community life of church potlucks. What was missing was any education about the primal instincts of the lower half of the body — of what could happen if I dropped into the "danger zone" of the scary unknown. I sensed that base emotions of anger and rage lived in these depths, and I didn't want to venture too far down for fear of them.

Body Myth 2 is fed by fear of the unknown and what it will bring if we venture outside of the comfort zone of our known world. This myth is also fed constantly because of the way our brains are wired. The neural circuits for survival — which look for anything possibly dangerous — fire much faster than the measured, thoughtful circuits that lead us into creative endeavors in new arenas.

To dispel this myth, the key is to slow down and expand our awareness — widen our perceptual lens on the world. Then we won't automatically decide that what might be a magic wand or a walking cane is always a dangerous snake! This becomes more nuanced as we take a closer look at all the ways the world can harm us and all the ways it can delight us.

Thawing Out the Freezer

I had worked with Janet for a number of months on her fear of relationships with men. What emerged, as she felt safe enough to share, was a particular memory that had haunted her for years.

When she was growing up, she had a beloved uncle who had always been her protector. He was her "listening ear" in a chaotic, alcoholic extended-family home. Unknown to her at the time, he still lived in their home because of his lifelong struggle with bipolar disorder and drug addiction.

One night, at age thirteen, Janet came home excited to share that she had gotten a big role in the school play. She rushed into her uncle's semidarkened room and gently shook his shoulder to wake him. He startled from his drug-induced stupor. Raging like a bull, he started to throttle her. The long seconds it took for him to recognize her and remove his hands from her throat seemed like an eternity. For her, it was a dreadful nightmare.

When the uncle finally let go, Janet fled from his room in shock and cried herself to sleep. Typical of many victims of violence, she took on the blame. Feeling ashamed, she hid the bruises that emerged on her neck with scarves and turtleneck sweaters so no one would know. Not only was she physically traumatized; she had lost her best friend.

Janet's sweet, quiet uncle became a monster in her eyes. She was not sure how it had happened, but she believed that somehow it was her fault. Perhaps it was her joy and exuberance that had ignited the rage deep within him. Perhaps *she* was responsible for this mysterious, life-threatening violence.

When her uncle awakened the next morning, he had no conscious memory of the incident. His addiction deepened in the weeks that followed. Soon after, he committed suicide, magnifying Janet's trauma, guilt, and shame. She walked around in a fog feeling like a zombie.

It was years before she could look fully at a man she cared about. If she was in a darkened room or a car at night with a man, her belly would grip in fear and her heart would pound, causing a panic attack. She was sure that something about her might cause men to turn into raging beasts. She withdrew further and further into herself.

As an adult, Janet finally went to psychotherapy and got the courage to ask remaining family members about her uncle. She discovered the truth about his lifelong struggles. This lessened her panic attacks, but she could not shake her deep mistrust of men and the sense that something about her might elicit a mysterious, dangerous rage from their depths.

CranioSacral Therapy and Dialogue

Body Myth 2 was alive and well in Janet's psyche and her nervous system. To dispel this myth, I sat with her and suggested that she needed a strong ally to meet this powerful fear. I asked her what would help her to feel more present with her thirteen-year-old self, who had made such an isolating decision to withdraw and protect herself.

She intuitively felt that, since this trauma was physically induced, she needed to be physically touched for this trauma to resolve. She also realized that she needed her wise adult self — the part of her that had done years of therapy — to be available to support her traumatized self. She was shaky but resolved as we began her session on my treatment table using my primary mode of hands-on healing, CranioSacral Therapy.

I gently let one of my hands hold the top of her chest while the other held her upper back, cradling her heart, as she recalled that night, first running up the stairs to share her joy with her uncle. I felt a trembling from her lower limbs that slowly dissipated.[1] Then I began to feel her chest tighten and get still and cold as she got closer to the actual traumatic moment. I let her know in a gentle voice that I was with her, as an ally, and that the grown-up part of her, who had uncovered the truth about her uncle, was also with us.

Janet's inner thirteen-year-old remained frozen and mute. Her chest continued to feel tight and cold. I let her know that I would patiently wait with her, as long as it took, for her to feel warmth there again.[2] I also reminded her that her cellular intelligence knew what to do and that she could let things unfold in her own time. Something shifted under my hands ever so slightly when I spoke. My words and presence conveyed to her that I saw her clearly, I was not pushing her, and I had no agenda about how this might unfold.

As I felt a deep stirring in her system, I explained that her frozenness was a natural nervous system response to such danger and that it had been her only possible defense at the time of her trauma. The numbness had helped her to survive such an overwhelming event. We explored whether she might want to thank it for its years of valiant service. I felt more stirring under my hands in response to those words.

Out of the Deep Freeze and into the Light of Awareness

It is often a surprising but welcome idea that we can have gratitude for a part of ourselves that was helpful in the past but is hindering our forward progress in the present moment.

Janet's chest softened significantly in the minutes that followed. This disowned part of herself, which had contributed to her panic attacks and mistrust of men, was finally feeling recognized for its original job of saving her from the overwhelming confusion, fear, and pain of the tragic experience with her uncle. With that recognition, the frozen tightness was able to loosen up a bit, slowly releasing its position as guardian of her safety.

I asked Janet's older, wiser self to explain to her thirteen-year-old self what had happened that night. Janet told her that it was not her exuberance and joy that had triggered her uncle's rage. It was not her fault at all. At the time of the event, he was deep in his own pain, confusion, and addiction, and she simply had no way of knowing that.

The older, wiser part of Janet thanked the freeze response, and I felt her chest coldness melt under my hands. Her breathing deepened and returned to normal as she cried sweet tears of relief.

In the aftermath of this session, Janet's panic attacks went away completely. She slowly began to make friends with the men in her life, at work and play. Her irrational sense of fear dissolved. That fear of her body and its panic response, as well as the fear of a primal rage response from men, was gone.

Body Myth 3: The Body Is Seductive and Leads You Astray

This body myth says that the *primal sensual and sexual urges* of the body will get us into trouble and lead us astray if we listen to and act on them.

Most major religions — whether Catholic, Protestant, Hindu, Muslim, and so on — impose sanctions against fully feeling the body so that this feared primal energy is kept in check. This is expressed in instructions like these:

"Guard against your body's urges."
"Control your body's impulses and sublimate them."
"Stay in charge of your body and hold its compulsions
    at bay."

Meanwhile, popular culture, advertising, and the media flood us with sexual images because marketers recognize that this primal energy can help sell almost anything. Advertisements turn around and twist what is acceptable and attractive, leaving most of us chasing a phantom image that promises to make us feel whole and lovable if only we buy into it.

In the meantime, the message is, "Whatever you do, do not fully feel your sensuality and sexuality — it is dangerous. If you are a woman, you might be preyed upon or called a *woman of loose morals*. If you are a man, you could be seen as *a dangerous predator.*"

This primal life force *is* powerful. My friend Emilie Conrad, who developed Continuum Movement,[3] taught that the energy of *eros*, the Greek word for "intimate love," is what makes our cells ignite. It allows us to feel our juiciness. In fact, it is the creative force of life itself. It feeds our joy and raison d'être, our reason for being.

Yet, Body Myth 3 tries to convince us that our core sensuality and sexuality are evil, seductive forces. How did this body myth come into power?

The problem arises when we judge this part of ourselves as bad, corrupt, or wicked and try to compartmentalize and seal off this powerful energy from the rest of our system. This acts like an aerosol can in the sun or a restless volcano building internal pressure. Like the closing love scene in *Like Water for Chocolate*, where the long-repressed lovers finally consummate their relationship and go up in flames in the process, this myth tells us that our sensuality, allowed free rein, will set fire to our world, burning out of control.

In fact, when we allow pleasurable sensation to flow through our entire system with the wisdom of each part of us informing and integrating it, the powerful energy we feel is not a force for evil. It is the energy of life itself.

If I am feeling sexually attracted to someone, it does not mean that I need to act on it. However, if I hold my sensual nature tightly wrapped, it can become a seductive shadow side of who I am. When we allow our sensations to fill *all* of us, the direct experience of this connection has a deep and abiding integrity, not a seductive one.

Locked Out of Her Own Sensuality

Karen is a high-powered administrator who successfully leads thousands of students at a major university. She came to see me with multiple physical issues that included asthma, chronic throat infections, and ongoing tightness in her solar plexus area, which made it hard to breathe deeply most of the time. My inner knowing was drawn directly to the area of her respiratory diaphragm, so we started our session with my hands on the front and back of her lower rib cage.

The sensation between my hands was of a drawn-in-tight achy pain. I asked her to drop her awareness inside to explore this area of her body with me. I felt her system pull in even tighter as she turned her attention inward.

She described to me the sense of her torso being not available, or "closed for business," as she said. I asked her how long it had felt that way, and she started to cry.

She told me that she was married to a wonderful man and had a daughter she adored. Even so, four years earlier she had fallen in love with someone else. There was a strong sexual attraction. He was a dynamic person who awakened her sensual side as a woman. The affair was short-lived, ending soon after her husband became aware of it. Feeling guilty, she shared that, when this happened, "I locked down my heart and pelvis and threw away the key."

She had spent the last four years struggling with her health and trying to prove to her husband that she still loved him and that she wanted the marriage to last. In her misguided fear that her core sensuality had caused the affair, she disconnected from the juiciest parts of who she was — and her health was suffering for it.

On my table she realized that she was afraid to breathe deeply or she might start to feel the "sensations" in her pelvis again. She said, "That was a primary part of what led me into the affair." Another key facet of self-blame, particularly for many women, is that when we find deep joy in our sensual experiences, it feels like a forbidden treasure, rather than one of our most primary natural responses.

She also had not forgiven herself for her "transgressions" and was carrying a heavy weight of guilt, which closed down her heart, slowing her energy flow further. Her throat was shut down as well, so she would not speak "the truth of my heart," she said.

I gently held her solar plexus and heart and asked what she would say if this affair had happened to her best friend. She got quiet and replied that she would feel compassion and would tell her friend to let go of her guilt and move on. I asked her if she could be her own best friend in that moment. I felt her body relax a bit as she took a deep breath and accepted that idea.

I then asked her if she was still in love with the other man, and if she wanted to leave her marriage. She said no; that moment in time had passed and she had moved on in her life. Another wave of relief released under my hands as she realized she was not in danger of succumbing to the seduction of this affair again.

As a woman living in our culture where sensuality is ignored or vilified, Karen's longing for a deep sensual connection made her vulnerable. A strong sexual attraction is almost impossible to refuse unless the integrity of the whole body is onboard.

I shared with Karen about the wisdom she could experience when her sensuality was alive and connected to all the other parts of her body. With the heart connected to the pelvis, gut, and head, we are inspired to approach important choices in our life journey by pausing, taking a breath, and seeing the bigger picture.

We realize the implications and probable end result of our choice. Our decisions become grounded and based on whole-body informed thinking.

We talked about recognizing that her natural, primal needs deserved to be fulfilled and that she could bring her sensual longing home as a gift to herself and her husband. This choice would validate Karen's grounded, whole-body-informed thinking.

Her torso relaxed slowly and completely as we spoke. She could sense that I held no judgment of her, had no agenda for her. Her sensual nature had not seduced her — it was not at fault.

We spent some time connecting her heart to her gut, her feet, and her legs, and then to the clarity of her bones and her head. When she got up off the table, the color had returned to her face. She was visibly more relaxed and present. Karen was awed by the depth of the work she had just done.

Karen is not alone in having this split between her head and her body. Body Myth 3 is alive and well in our culture, and many powerful women have left their body behind to get the job done successfully. This split creates vulnerability and makes us susceptible to the pulls and tugs of sensations that are only seductive in isolation.

Body Myth 4: The Body Is Out of Control and Must Be Dominated

Do you see your body as something you have to constantly control — masterfully riding it until it gives you what you want? This myth about the body centers around the idea that *if you are not controlling it in every moment*, your body will become something despicable, or it will collapse emotionally and fall apart. So you work to control it, altering it in whatever ways you think will get you love and acceptance, as well as safety and protection from harm. It is a fact that to feel loved and accepted is a primary human need, so fear of losing this feeds Body Myth 4.

For instance, you may discipline yourself to diet and exercise, not as an act of loving self-care, but rather in an attempt to create the body you think will make you more lovable, safe, or protected.

This form of self-judgment about your body may be based on cultural norms, the media, or friends and family. To have an acceptable body, you may feel you have to live your life on a diet or constantly work out. Controlling what you eat in this way and pushing your body physically beyond healthy limits are both natural outcomes of believing Body Myth 4.

At a deeper level, this body myth may be fueled by unresolved trauma. If you have a history of feeling overwhelmed by traumatic events, then the alarm bells of the nervous system may continue to sound in your head and body long after an event has ended. In general, the external world may feel overwhelming and out of control. This could, in turn, cause you to exert extreme control over the areas of your life that you *can* control.

Witnessing the effects of pain and trauma in others can also be traumatizing. Consider the high number of people who suffer from post-traumatic stress disorder (PTSD) after witnessing a terrorist act.

If, when you were a child, someone you loved wailed and cried uncontrollably whenever they felt emotionally overwhelmed, as an adult you might find that similar sounds put you into an alarm state. You might become hypervigilant even though you are not personally in danger. You could find your insides going numb, the way you did as a child, to control your own fearful feelings.

All of the above can be a huge impetus to clamp down and control the body and its reactions to a life that seems threatening.

Control at All Costs

James came sauntering into my office with his clean-cut good looks, muscular physique, and big smile masking his deep pain and anxiety.

It did not take long for his pain to surface, first reported as numbness. "I can't feel what you are talking about in my body. I have no idea what you are asking me to do or feel," James reported to me.

When I asked him what his childhood was like, James sarcastically replied that it was "normal." He was the eldest of three boys. When his dad would come home from work, his mother would report the antics of his sons that day, and his father would discipline them by *sticking their heads in the toilet and flushing it.* When I asked how that abuse had affected him, James displayed his degree of self-judgment by saying, "What abuse? We deserved it — we were really bad."

Upon further inquiry, it became apparent that James was echoing what his father had said to them. James was quite certain that he had not been a good child and that his father had "only been trying to keep me in line."

James described how he had spent his life trying to please his overly critical father, who was so self-centered that he never really knew James or his other sons. This is codependence on steroids. His father was an alcoholic who drank at night and took his inner angst out on his sons, physically and emotionally. This had taken a heavy toll on James, who had a huge tender heart battered by years of abuse.

By his fifteenth birthday, James was as tall as his father. One evening when his dad came home drunk and started to abuse his younger brother, James ended up pinning his dad to the wall. That was the last time his dad hit anyone in the family. He stopped drinking shortly thereafter, but his inability to show love to his sons continued.

James was in his early thirties when he came to see me. He was a Navy SEAL who had hardened his body through grueling workouts and training. He rarely visited his parents, so dealing with his father was no longer the problem. What plagued him was that he was unable to let his tenderness emerge in his marriage and with his own children, and he desperately wanted that.

Whenever James had a difference of opinion with his wife or kids, and his emotions began to surface, he felt threatened. His body response was to go numb and withdraw. If pushed further, he would become enraged. This scared everyone, including James.

James did not want to reenact his own childhood, and yet he felt helpless and out of control of his body and mind. In those situations, his emotions seemed to belong to someone else. He tried to keep himself under control by working out relentlessly every day. After an especially hard workout, he would come home tired and finally sleep well at night.

I began our sessions by asking him to take his awareness inside, to follow his breath and let it deepen as he felt his entire body all the way to his feet on the floor. For weeks he practiced the basic inner-awareness exercise (see chapter 4, "Exploration 1: Opening Awareness," pages 55–59), but all he felt was continuing numbness.

All James's Navy SEAL discipline came in handy, since he stuck with it, week after week. I asked him to be patient and keep returning his awareness within, simply being kind and not judging. I asked him to act toward himself the way he would with his best buddy.

After several months of this daily practice, the numbness started to change. His purposeful yet nonjudgmental attention to inner sensations, no matter how uncomfortable or downright painful they might be, was paying off.

He was learning to cultivate his curiosity, his openness to discovery, rather than his habitual pattern of clamping down on all feelings and sensations. James was building his capacity to be with himself, no matter what showed up in his awareness.

Then we moved to the next stage, where James allowed himself to fill up with nurturing sensation, creating an inner container of nourishment for himself that helped him feel stronger and steadier. His numbness was dissipating layer by layer as he felt fuller and fuller.

With a steady container of sensation to depend on, James felt safe enough to have issues surface. Initially, all he felt was a general muscular tension throughout his body, as though he were tightening down for protection or preparing to run.

Then actual early memories began to surface. We worked through them together, holding and cradling the tender abused little boy that he had been. Slowly, James came to understand that he had not been a bad child at all. Finally, he recognized himself for the sensitive, caring brother that he was. His sadness emerged, and his tears flowed freely.

Within that strong, fit, man-body was a little boy who was still defending himself against the blows of his father, from whom he only wanted love.

The painstaking process of teaching James to feel his own body again, without immediately rushing in to control it, required my patience and willingness to move at a careful, purposeful pace that worked for him. We could only move as fast as the slowest part of him felt safe to go.

Initially, James could not relax and turn off the fight-or-flight response. Feeling *anything* would set him off. In those moments I would help him to slow his process so as to grow a greater sense of grounding and build a bigger, stronger container to hold his emotions.

As the months passed, he developed trust in the process. As he continued the daily practice of calming himself and dropping inside to explore his feelings, James eventually began to have a different experience. He was recognizing that it was paying off.

His wife remembered why she had fallen in love with him. Once again, James was able to see her and his children for the wonderful human beings they were.

Even though there was occasional backsliding into the old behaviors, this happened less and less, and James's huge heart and loving tenderness emerged to the delight of those in his world.

James told me about his fellow SEALs and how he could now sense their pain and woundedness. I suggested that he sit with them and simply listen if they needed to talk.

He would grin at me and say, "If they could see me now, crying and admitting that I have such a big tender heart!" We laughed together, and I knew he was on his way home to himself and that Body Myth 4 no longer had him in its grip.

With up to one-third of our current population suffering from the effects of past trauma, learning to heal in this way is paramount for everyone. Doing so will change the trajectory of the lineage we unknowingly hand down to our children or inflict upon our partners and community.

In the attachment research world, Dr. Daniel Siegel names having a "coherent narrative" about one's childhood as the biggest predictor of whether a traumatic attachment history will get unknowingly passed on to one's children.[4] A coherent narrative requires self-awareness and enough healing about our own childhood and attachment experience to be able to recognize and avoid repeating it with our own children.

This is hopeful because it says we can change the unconscious patterns of how we connect or not with those closest to us. Healing in this way also frees us up to manifest the gifts we were born to share with the world.

Body Myth 5: The Body Knows Far Less Than the Brain

I am continually mystified by the brilliant minds I know who second-guess their instinctual gut knowing, or their heart's inspiration, or their bones' deep clarity, and as a result drive themselves crazy. Most of us in the Western world are trained to trust our logical left brain and rational thoughts over our body.

In the last decade neuroscience has shown that the gut (or the enteric nervous system, which is called our "second brain") makes *more* neurotransmitters than the brain that resides in our head.[5] I recently read astounding research showing that *the body registers incoming events before the mind or visual system can see them coming.*[6] Many of us remember circumstances when our body took a wise action that saved us before our mind had time to react.

And yet, Body Myth 5 remains epidemic in our culture, which I will be talking about in more detail throughout this book. The late Emilie Conrad, my wonderful colleague and friend, used to say, "Admit it, Suzanne. We in the bodywork and movement fields are still out in the barn. The rest of academia is up in the mansion discussing the future of humanity, and if we are honest, we are still out in the barn with the animals because of our focus on the wisdom of the body."

It is time to move out of the barn! Again and again, I see evidence of the split between the wisdom of the body and the logical brain. This lack of understanding of our body wisdom wreaks havoc on our health and well-being and robs us of our potential for happiness and the juiciness and joy inherent in life.

Our bodies are naturally well-calibrated navigational systems once we learn how to listen to them and respect their assessments in any given moment. If we disrespect our bodies and second-guess their messages, they will go mute over time. The loss of our body wisdom leaves us vulnerable, as we are forced to navigate our life with only the signals from the brain and past experiences.

It is our *present-moment sensory experience* that provides the foundational data to the prefrontal area of our brain for the wisest decision-making possible. Without a conscious *sensory* connection to the present, we are forced to orient to the past.

People with unresolved trauma histories are at an even

greater disadvantage due to numb, frozen, and painful places in their bodies, keeping them from accessing this wisdom.

Amazed and Dazed

Bartholomew is a brilliant physician and an excellent pediatrician whose mind has served him well. When he first entered my world, he was looking for answers to leg pain that had plagued him for years.

During our initial interview, I realized he was looking for a medical, left-brain reason for why his pain persisted even though his allopathic medical worldview had failed to explain it.

In his first craniosacral session, I tuned in to his body's wisdom and gently took his leg and foot in my hands. He felt a growing shakiness inside, in the area between my two hands. As he tuned in to the exact area of his leg pain, things got even shakier and his leg started visibly trembling.

In order to help him understand what was happening, I briefly explained Dr. John Upledger's "energy cyst" model, which describes how trauma memory in the form of disorganized, chaotic energy is walled off and encapsulated in the body in order to help the system deal with things that are overwhelming at the time of the trauma.[7] I explained that when the time is right, the body naturally wants to let go of this chaotic energy so that it can function better again. I further reassured him that this is a natural body release process, so he could understand and relax into the shakiness and the other sensations that were occurring.

An actual memory surfaced about an accident that had occurred a decade earlier. While Bartholomew rested during a hike in a remote canyon out West, a huge branch fell, glanced off his head, and landed on his leg. He was in shock initially, and others helped to lift off the heavy branch. Bartholomew worried that he had broken his leg because the impact was so powerful, but in the end, he was okay and could hike out of the canyon on his own. He had long since left this incident behind, but his leg had not.

Bartholomew was slightly dazed and totally amazed! The trembling and release from his leg was undeniable. He felt ripples of new awareness enter him as the pain left his leg. When we were done, his pain level was significantly reduced, and it continued to drop.

When Bartholomew arrived for his next visit, his analytical mind was back in the driver's seat. Even though he was still free from pain, he was second-guessing his experience. His left brain had once again taken over and his body's wisdom had gone mute. I reminded him of exactly what had occurred in our session. It was as though he had amnesia about the process. It certainly did not fit any model he had studied in medical school.

I realized that he needed more body awareness, more inner-sensation experiences, to overcome this prejudice, so I taught him the Core Embodiment Process that I have been refining for years (see Exploration 2, pages 59–66). Bartholomew has now been doing this body-centered practice for several years. He no longer immediately questions his body's wisdom. However, he still relies on his mind to corroborate what he is feeling, just to make sure it is real.

Wisdom Ignored at a Price

When Cassie arrived at my office, she was suffering with relentless shin and leg pain. She had recently run in a marathon, and in the second half of the race, her knees and shins had started to ache. She mistakenly thought, if she continued to run, her endorphins would take care of the problem. Instead, it grew steadily worse.

Cassie did not listen to her body but plowed on, letting her mind's agenda override the obvious pain message telling her to stop. By the time she reached the finish line, Cassie was hobbling, and she had been hobbling ever since.

As we worked together, it became apparent that one of the reasons Cassie was not healing was because she was "angry with my stupid body for not doing what I wanted it to do." Further, she was not giving her legs the rest they needed in order to heal due to her anger and frustration about how they *should* be behaving.

In her CranioSacral Therapy session, I held her shins and knees and tuned in to what was going on. The initial sensations under my hands felt really hot and inflamed. I asked her what she noticed when she dropped her attention down into her legs.

Cassie had a hard time getting there at first, but then she registered shock as she began to feel the heat. I explained to her that when tissue is inflamed like hers, no amount of willpower can heal the area if the person is not prepared to work with the body's wisdom about what it needs.

Cassie went silent for a few minutes, and then she shared how her Asian immigrant family lineage was one of pushing through and beyond the needs of the body in order to survive. Willing herself to do more, go beyond, and not listen to her body was all she knew.

In Cassie's family, the body was seen as the servant to the mind, whose sole purpose was to further the family and individual standing in their community. This attitude is almost epidemic in our culture today in many ethnic groups.

As I continued to hold her legs, she slowly allowed herself to recognize how her family belief system was impeding her healing process. We dialogued with her legs, and she made a promise to allow them to rest and heal, demonstrating how she valued them. She was able to see that resting did not equal weakness, but it actually was a sign of intelligence — body intelligence, that is.

Within weeks, her legs were well on their way to healing after months of inflammation and pain. With that, Body Myth 5 was dispelled. Cassie was hopefully on her way to greater body wisdom in the rest of her life as well.

Where Do We Go from Here?

These five body myths, or some combination, are alive and well in many people today. Take a moment now and consider which of these are hindering your life.

Awareness is the first step in letting go of them and making a new choice. Until we are aware that they are playing in the background or foreground of our lives, often driving our actions and decisions, we will be unable to choose anything different.

Of course, the second part of this equation is recognizing them as myths. *These attitudes are not a part of our true nature.* They are adaptations, compensations, and defenses against what has occurred in our lives and those of our ancestors.

When we can recognize these myths for what they truly are — myths — new horizons open up. New choices can be made. We are free to be who we are at a deeper, more authentic level. Then life is experienced at a richer level with more joy, more ease, more realness, and all that entails. Life does not become a rose garden, but it has more resonance with who we truly are at a soul level.

3 The Hallmarks of Optimum Health

Finding the Path Home

> *To love oneself is the beginning of a lifelong romance.*
>
> — OSCAR WILDE

As we travel through the systems of our body, learning to listen to and use its wisdom, we would be wise to be on the lookout for the signs of optimum health — the road maps that lead us in the right direction.

One of the hallmarks of a healthy system is appropriate and constant connection between all of its parts. When you have an optimal flow of information throughout, it supports the life of your system, creating a feeling of well-being and balance.

Healthy Boundaries and Healthy Connections

At a micro level, the same principles of healthy boundaries and healthy connections apply. Existing within a membrane, all our cells operate in constant communication with one another. Every healthy cell continuously receives oxygen and releases carbon dioxide, allowing life-giving nutrients in and keeping toxic substances out.

A vigorous immune system is consistently providing us with protection from the pathogens in our environment.

At a macro level, these principles are also true. A strong family unit provides safety, stability, love, and nurturing to all its members. In this secure atmosphere, we develop trust that when our needs arise, they can and will be met.

When organizations are healthy, they operate in a manner that supports the individuals within the system, the mission of the institution, and the greater world.

What Goes Wrong?

So what happens to us as human beings? Beginning in utero and throughout our lives, each of us has experiences that are less than optimal. This may be a persistent condition, such as poverty or chronic ill health, or it may be just the everyday stressful issues related to work and family. The fact is everyone experiences daily events that are traumatizing in small and sometimes large ways.

When our body senses a threat, we instinctively take action to protect ourselves. We tighten down and hunch our shoulders. Our hearts beat faster, and our breathing gets shallower. Our spines may compress, causing neck and back pain. We may stumble or fall as we rush to get somewhere.

We anxiously yell at someone who may be the object of our fear or frustration, and that person may yell back at us! All of this protective behavior results in cycles of tension and pain as we tighten our gut, curl in our shoulders, grip our tailbone, and clench our jaw. This is the body's attempt to protect us from possible harm and prepare us to perhaps fight or flee.

Then there are the ordinary, "under the radar" traumas we don't recognize as such. These "small" things don't seem like much at the time, but we react to them in ways that mold our future. Rather than minimize this kind of trauma, I want to emphasize the importance of it, even though we are often unaware of it at the time. The impact can be profound and chronic if this kind of trauma is not processed and healed.

For example, Tony is a caring nurse practitioner who manages a team of hospice nurses. He always appears calm, unflappable, and caring. He volunteers, stays late, has extra degrees, is impeccably groomed, and is soft spoken. He has set three dates to retire, and each time he has decided to stay on. Recently, he came in for a session after having a heart attack.

Lying on the treatment table, he remembered standing at the top of the stairs in his childhood home, listening to his single mother on the phone. His younger brother had broken his arm again, and his mother didn't know how she was going to pay the doctor's bills or how she could miss work to stay home with the boy.

Tony became aware that that was the moment he decided he would give up everything to make sure his mother didn't worry: He volunteered to stay home with his brother, made sure the house was always clean, and kept straight As in school. His whole life became dedicated to caring for others, but ultimately at his own expense.

This seemingly small decision made in early childhood created a mandate that was still operating decades later — and wreaking havoc on his health. Stories like Tony's show up in my classes and practice constantly — seemingly "small" decisions can affect the whole direction of our lives, or the pace we keep, or the people we choose to be in relationship with, and so on.

New Research on Trauma

In the last decade, exciting research on trauma has been coming in from all directions. These studies point to how human mental disorders, chronic pain and illness, and even everyday tension can come as a direct result of unresolved past trauma. Bessel van der Kolk and many others have looked at populations at risk and the number of psychiatric diagnoses (such as bipolar, oppositional-defiant disorder, ADHD, and so on) whose roots most likely grow out of traumatic experiences.[1]

In the 1990s, the "Adverse Childhood Experiences Study," conducted by the Centers for Disease Control and Prevention (CDC) and Kaiser Permanente, looked at physical and mental health in middle-aged adults when early childhood experiences were threatening, negative, or damaging in some way.[2] They surveyed seventeen thousand patients from 1995 to 1997, and these found that adults with a significant number of adverse childhood experiences had significantly impaired health and adult functioning on all levels. The CDC continues to follow these patients, so the longitudinal data is still being gathered.

Let's take a look at how this manifests.

Daily Tension and Acute Trauma

As I have described, when something adverse happens, our systems naturally tighten down and go into a protective state. When the threat or danger passes, *ideally* we realize this and release the tension. After a long, harried commute, being able to relax and walk in the door ready to start our workday would be optimal. Unfortunately, most of us forget to stop, take a deep breath, and relax our neck and shoulders. Instead, we carry the tension from the drive right into our offices, which is not a good way to start the day.

Consider Sally, who experienced a significant emotional trauma prior to coming to work. Sally's beloved cat died after a long night at the vet's office, and she had an important meeting early the next morning. Sally felt sadness and a heavy heart over her pet's death, but these emotions had no place in her business meeting. So she held in her emotions and contained her sadness throughout the day. When Sally finally got home, she had a splitting headache and was too exhausted to allow her true feelings to come to the surface and be expressed.

When the event is a serious physical injury due to a car accident, a fall, a head injury, or any painful trauma to the body, the body's first response is shock, the ultimate protective state. Shock can manifest as numbness or paralysis. Often, the pain does not register until the shock has dissipated. Only then can the body's work of healing itself begin. The effects of this level of trauma can last for years depending on the severity of the injury and the level of attention it receives.

Chronic Harmful Experiences

People can also carry a *chronic* level of tension in their body from adverse childhood experiences, such as physical and emotional abuse or neglect, a parent with mental illness, or an environment that does not feel safe due to violence or drug use.[3] To an abused child who feels overwhelmed and frozen, the trauma may be experienced simply as pain, numbness, or disconnection.

In order to survive and continue to function, the body will encapsulate and wall off the effect of the trauma (per Dr. John Upledger's energy cyst model, which I mention in chapter 2). This compartmentalization is often outside the child's conscious awareness. They may feel emotionally flat, their system muted. Unable to experience normal emotional responses to everyday, ordinary events, they may act out, attacking themselves or others, as though their body is trying to rid itself of the trauma in any way possible.

Of course, people can experience a combination of chronic and acute trauma. A sadly repeated example of this tragedy is chronic childhood abuse followed by an event that causes PTSD, such as the acute physical and emotional injuries that soldiers suffer while in a war zone. A landmark longitudinal Harvard study showed clearly that those without trauma histories can eventually recover from the horror of war, while those who also suffer from childhood traumatic experiences may still experience painful, incapacitating PTSD symptoms, such as nightmares, flashbacks, and dissociation, even after fifty years.[4] The experiences of war cause prior defenses from childhood trauma to be refortified and locked even more deeply into the system, making it doubly difficult to heal in the aftermath.

The Effect of Blocked Trauma in the Body

If optimal health is where the entire system is constantly communicating, internally and externally, what happens when the effects of trauma become lodged in the tissues of the body?

In a healthy system, the body responds by sending immune system resources to the site of the injury or trauma, instigating a healing response. There is a specific walling off of the area so that it can heal while containing the effects of the damage. This is followed by a timely reintegration when the healing is complete.

However, if the disturbance is physically or emotionally overwhelming and doesn't resolve in an advantageous way, the body will create an ever-stronger container for the damage.

In *When the Body Says No*, Gabor Maté addresses the long-term issues, "the price we pay," when unresolved trauma continues to fester for decades.[5] His research and clinical observations have shown that many of our chronic illnesses may have early trauma or current traumatic events as their root cause. This includes autoimmune diseases such as MS, lupus, scleroderma, and other debilitating disorders.

When our bodies hold on to trauma — physically, emotionally, or mentally — the healthy give-and-take of our cells is impaired. How long this effect lasts and what is required for healing depends on many factors, but the good news is that it *is* repairable. This book is designed to teach you how to stimulate the repair process and show you how to get back into the driver's seat of your "bus of health."

Experiencing the Present Moment Requires Safety and Connection

One of the consequences of unresolved trauma is the way in which it locks people out of an accurate assessment of what is actually happening in any given moment. Present-moment awareness is very tough if not impossible for those haunted by past memories (or flashbacks) and plagued by constant anxiety of the future. When the very navigational system that provides information about the present moment is impaired, frozen, or captivated by trauma memories, people miss the signals that tell them danger is approaching or that they could make a certain choice because it feels "right."

This means our first step in reclaiming our cells (and ourselves) is to return to the present moment — and we must feel safe in order to do that. "Be in the present moment" is an excellent mandate, but without a sense of physical and emotional safety, it is extremely challenging.

The research of Dr. Stephen Porges shows us clearly that the vagus nerve is the core signal giver in our parasympathetic nervous system regarding safety and a sense of healthy connection.[6] He clearly establishes that this system, so elegant and automatic when operating optimally, is severely impaired in trauma survivors and other at-risk populations.

His findings back up my clinical and classroom experiences. Over the last three decades, these experiences have fueled my quest for better ways to help people have more present-moment full-body sensations.

An internal felt sense of *safety* and *connection* clearly is a pivotal need for all of us as we reclaim our body and come home to ourselves more fully in each present moment of our lives.

However, the question then becomes, what paths are most effective for establishing a sense of safety and of healing, nurturing connection?

The most effective approach I have found is nurturing touch: professionally through CranioSacral Therapy, and personally with warm hugs and other physical affection.

Talking about Touch

Nurturing touch is a primary way that we know who we are and where we are as human beings. When we are touched in a safe, nourishing way, we become more aware of what is actually going on in the present moment. There are decades of research on how appropriate touch from birth onward increases physical resilience, health, intelligence, and creativity.[7]

When I am on the treatment table with a good practitioner, I can access sensations and inner wisdom previously outside of my awareness. Excellent bodywork of all kinds helps us feel more of who we are in the best sense.

I love the following quote by Dr. Bessel van der Kolk, a psychiatrist who is now a major proponent of touch therapies for healing trauma.

> Touch helped me enormously. Touch had been strictly prohibited in my training and sorely neglected in my upbringing, but...touch helped me become more aware of my inner experiences and made me understand the enormous power of touch to help people borrow comfort and physiological safety from each other.
>
> Becoming aware of inner sensations, our primordial feelings, allows us access to the direct experience of our own living body.[8]

That direct experience of our own living body is vital for healing, no matter the cause of our distress. Now that we have an improved understanding of human trauma, and appreciate the role of proper therapeutic support, our healing process can be more efficient and enjoyable.

I'm excited to share what I've learned about the wisdom centers of the body, about how every area of who we are has its own unique knowing. The whispers of your heart are distinct from the knowing of your gut. The power of your pelvis is grounded by the clarity in your bones and activated by the metabolizing talent of your legs and feet. Harnessing all that wisdom, and combining it with a flexible and integrative brain, will help you live life more fully.

In chapters 5 through 10, we dive into the main wisdom areas of the body — the heart, gut, pelvis, legs and feet, bones, and brain — and explore their unique roles in the process of developing full-body presence. We'll also discover how, when we are operating optimally, all of these areas are in connection and communication with one another. Sometimes, our main obstacle to healing is that one wisdom area is mistakenly trying to "go it alone" — soldiering solo through life's challenges, when the rest of the team is standing by, ready to work together.

The next chapter sets the stage for exploring our body's wisdom areas by presenting ways to experience direct sensation. Developing this skill is necessary to be able to hear the messages of your body.

4

Embodying Fully
Practices to Live By

and i said to my body. softly. 'i want to be your friend.'
it took a long breath. and replied 'i have been waiting
my whole life for this.'

— NAYYIRAH WAHEED

This chapter presents three practices, or explorations, that readers of my first book, *Full Body Presence*, will recognize as old friends.[1] These cultivate the skill set you need to deepen your embodiment process and practice actually experiencing your inner landscape. Conceptual knowledge alone is no substitute for direct experience.

The linear mind tends to discount this process because it is so simple. However, do not be deceived. This process has profound implications for the quality of how you experience your life. It will bring a richness and depth to your inner awareness — to your awakening consciousness — that is vital. Our mental faculties may be able to conceive of this process, but from one step removed. I invite you to step into this big, gentle river, not just watch from the banks.

My first three explorations are based on the understanding

that the earth's field is our foundation and a core resource for our physical bodies. Who we are and how our cells are formed and function is all in relationship to the earth and its gravitational field. Inner awareness, mindfulness, is vital, but unless we recognize the larger field within which we exist, we run the risk of becoming isolated from the steady and nourishing resource that is available as long as we are alive.

In addition, each of the six "wisdom area" chapters has its own dedicated exploration, and taken together, they merge the senses of your heart, gut, pelvis, legs and feet, bones, and brain into a unified, integrated, potent single system — you. This will offer you depth and richness in your direct experience of being alive.

This chapter's three explorations are as follows:

1. **Opening Awareness:** Exploration 1 focuses on how present you are *first* before any intentions are set, other than simple and deep listening — noticing any signals or information that your inner landscape may have for you from this neutral place.

2. **The Core Embodiment Process:** Exploration 2 grounds and fills the container of who you are with nourishing, nurturing sensation. This process allows you to mindfully and purposefully offer each cell of your being sensations that nourish you at a core level.

3. **Healing the Internal Resistance to Life:** Exploration 3 is where you learn to integrate those places that are still feeling disconnected within. We all have them. Knowing how to come back into oneness and integration with those disconnected pockets of who we are, in a gentle yet powerful and loving manner, is a vital skill for life itself.

Even if you have read my first book and are well practiced in the three foundational explorations that follow, I suggest you read the refinements I have added to the directions or "how-to" instructions below. Over the last twenty-five years, I've discovered many subtle enhancements and understandings that assist the process of staying in the present moment of direct sensation experience — all of which deepen the practice significantly for me. May they be of help to you as well.

If you are new to these explorations, I suggest you read the instructions closely and practice all three explorations. These lay the foundation for an optimal experience of the six wisdom areas and their individual meditations in the next chapters.

Finally, all the explorations in this book are available as audio files that you can download online. These audio explorations are central to this material. I've provided transcripts of these files for those who prefer to read the explorations or have difficulty with audio comprehension. However, once you've read the transcripts, I recommend practicing each exploration with the audio, which allows you to close your eyes and simply experience it. I have included download instructions throughout the book. To download the audio file of any exploration, go to www.healingfromthecore.com, click on the Reclaiming Your Body Download link, and enter the password *presence*.

How to Practice the Explorations

Find a good location: These practices work best if you find a quiet place where you will be undisturbed. For maximum effect, avoid or mute technology (other than what's needed for the audio exploration) and minimize environmental noise and intrusions by other people.

Special note: Do not listen to any of these explorations while driving a vehicle or operating heavy machinery, as they can lead listeners into a deep state of relaxed awareness and may cause drowsiness.

Keep your feet in contact with the ground: Sit comfortably, back supported, with the bottoms of your feet in contact with the ground beneath you. You can leave your shoes on if they are comfortable and allow for full contact with whatever is beneath you.

Special note: I spent almost two decades practicing meditation with my legs tucked up under me in full lotus position. What I discovered is that this position does not allow for easy movement of energy below the hips, so it is counterproductive when cultivating a sense of presence in your legs and feet.

For those who find sitting uncomfortable or distracting, these explorations can be done lying on your back with your knees bent and the bottoms of your feet flat on the floor (or whatever surface you are resting on). This position does more easily lead to falling asleep, so it is not ideal, but it can work. I have heard from many across the years who start their day with my explorations while lying in bed, with good results.

Keep your eyes closed or semiclosed: Entering the world of your inner landscape is best done when your visual system is mostly or completely quieted. If you tend to fall asleep when you close your eyes, allow them to be partially closed with a soft focus.

Special note: For those who fall asleep upon closing their eyes, adding gentle movement or touch helps keep the awareness parts of the brain from shutting off completely, which can lead to sleep. One way to do this is to lightly rub slow circles on your knees with your hands. Some prefer slowly running the palms gently up and down the outside of the thighs, which is another method that works.

Conceptual Preparation for the Explorations

Sensations are our building blocks: During the explorations, allow yourself to notice whatever basic sensations show up — temperature, texture, color, shape, weight, density, and symmetry. Notice these direct sensations without any interpretation — simple perceptions from your present-moment experience without a story. They are the alphabet of the language of your inner landscape.

For example, you may notice sensations along the spectrum of wet to dry and all temperatures, from hot, warm, or tepid to cool, cold, or even frozen. You may feel compressed and dense or spacious; loose or tight; heavy or light; sharp or dull; tingling, vibrating, humming, or pulsing; sparky and electric or smooth, calm, and quiet. If you are a visual person, you may see colors or get visual images — simply allow yourself to feel the sensations that the colors or images elicit, such as the warmth of the bright sun or the cool smoothness of silver. You may experience a range of taste sensations — such as sweet, bitter, salty, and so on — and of smells, such as fragrant, musty, or floral. Each person's experience will be completely unique, so if other sensations show up, welcome them. Your experience will also most likely change with time and practice.

It is important to register the sensation in your conscious awareness *without interpretation* — avoid stories that pull you into the past or the future. I call this level of awareness — which allows you to stay more easily in the *present moment of your immediate experience* — "deep informing."

If a story or an emotion arises, know that this frequently occurs and you are not alone. You have not done anything wrong. Simply drop to the layer below the emotional state into your direct-sensation experience.

By gently bringing yourself back into the immediate sensation, you prevent being pulled out of the moment and into the story that emotions often elicit. Be curious about the sensations underneath the emotion. For instance, grief might feel wet and heavy with dark-colored undertones. Anger may feel hot or cold; it may feel electric and look red. Gratitude may feel warm and spacious. Shame may feel tight or contracted with a warm wash of sensation to the face. Fear might feel constricted or buzzy, and so on. The possibilities are limitless!

Listen to the sensation response in your own body: Your inner landscape speaks to you through felt sensations, images, words heard internally, and other intuitive hits. As you listen to the audio of the exploration, allow yourself to simply notice and feel whatever shows up in that area of your body in response to my questions.

Go at your own pace: If you need to slow down in one area and take more time, do that. These explorations are simply leading you into the territory where your own inner wisdom can offer you deep informing of some kind. When that occurs, allow my voice to drop away and stay with whatever wisdom is informing you.

Spiritual Preparation for the Explorations

Three main attributes can lead you to a much deeper experience. I consider these spiritual preparation: curiosity, awareness, and trust.

Engage your curiosity: Let your judgmental mind take a rest. Simply be curious about new internal sensations, and stay open to new discoveries. This allows for breakthrough awareness to arise in the safety of a nonjudgmental attitude.

When you notice judgment trying to slip back in the door, and it most likely will (perhaps even multiple times!), simply recognize it and gently but firmly escort it out. Nothing pulls us out of the direct experience of present-moment consciousness like judgment, with its stories, rules, and emotionally charged conclusions about yourself, others, or the world.

Embrace present-moment awareness: Everything is simply information. Whatever direct sensations, internal hits, or "aha" moments come into your consciousness, simply welcome them, acknowledge them, and when you are ready, move on with as little judgment as possible.

Deep states of consciousness, what I call expanded awareness, can arise when you recognize that all time exists in the present moment. Anything you need from the future or whatever is relevant or needs healing from the past can be held in your awareness in the present moment.

Trust the process: As you engage your curiosity and embrace present-moment awareness, trusting the process augments the experience. The attribute of trust throws open the doors to endless possibilities for healthy, creative outcomes to life's most troublesome issues.

Many people have experienced traumas that can make it challenging to trust the present moment. However, rather than doing or thinking on automatic pilot (usually run by old fear-inducing experiences), know that when you trust your present-moment awareness and go at your own pace, the natural flow of life occurs with a lot more grace and ease.

With all of this in mind, download the audio (see instructions above) and practice each of the three foundational explorations that follow. They will give you an excellent general sense of your internal landscape. They are time tested and work beautifully when practiced regularly, and they will bring more meaning and resonance to each of the other body wisdom explorations in the following chapters. Enjoy!

EXPLORATION 1

Opening Awareness

Where Am I in This Moment?

Welcome to Exploration 1.

Begin by settling in, gliding into neutral, releasing your expectations, agendas, and judgments. Allow yourself to naturally, effortlessly respond to the following suggestions and questions, knowing that the ideal response is whatever spontaneously shows up in your body and your conscious awareness as we go. The nature of your experience will naturally change and deepen as this process unfolds and with repeated practice.

Choose a comfortable seat with good back support and let your feet rest easily and fully on the floor. Take a moment now to get comfortable, and then we'll begin.

[Pause]

As you close your eyes or partially close your eyes, turning your attention inward, gather your awareness, your openness to discovery, and let it travel in with your breath, following your inhalation down into your lungs...settling your conscious awareness inside your body — and letting the external world fall away.

Let's begin by taking a baseline reading, an overall look, inwardly scanning your entire body from head to toe, being curious about anything that pops into your awareness, noting areas that feel at ease, comfortable — in other words, where you feel more connection. You may notice sensations of warmth or coolness, a sense of fullness or spaciousness. Allow yourself to take in these sensations, no matter how subtle. Take a few moments now to notice any area or areas where you feel more sense of connection.

[Pause]

Then notice the internal areas that feel less present, where there is less sensation, or perhaps pain or numbness. Just notice without judgment. You may notice discomfort or a lack of feeling. Certain areas may simply feel more distant. Notice anywhere that you feel less connected right now. Internally scanning, relaxed.

You are taking a baseline sensory snapshot of how you feel overall as you begin.

[Pause]

Now bring your attention back to your breath and allow yourself to be curious about the subtle sensations of breathing. Notice the temperature of the air as it enters your nose and throat, traveling down into your lungs. Is it cool or warm? Feel the rise and fall of your ribs. Is there anywhere that your breathing feels restricted, or is it easy and full?

As you inhale and exhale, do you notice your chest rising and falling, or are you more aware of your back resting against the chair? In other words, is more of you present right now in the front of you or in the back? Or do you feel them both equally?

Allow your attention to move up into your neck and head. What do they feel like?

What do your eyes feel like? Is there any sense of strain or are they relaxed? How does the air around you feel on your cheeks?

What does your mouth feel like? Is your jaw tight or relaxed? How do your teeth and gums and tongue feel?

How does your neck feel right now? Does one side feel more relaxed than the other? How does your throat feel?

Returning to your chest, notice your breathing again for a moment. With your deepening awareness, do you notice any changes? How does the rise and fall of your ribs feel now?

How does your heart feel? Allow yourself to feel the sensations in your heart area with as little interpretation as possible. Can you feel it beating? Be aware of all the different ways you receive sensation. Does your heart feel like a particular color?

And letting your attention spread out from the heart area, allow yourself to notice the sensations in the rest of your chest …and on out to your shoulders…your upper back…down your arms into your hands and fingers. How do your arms and hands feel? Heavy or light? Distant or connected to your chest and heart? Pulsating or vibrating? How do your arms and hands feel right now?

When you are ready, allow your attention to return to your breath, letting your awareness drop down as you exhale, settling into your torso, deeper and wider with each exhale…simply noticing. Does one side of your torso feel denser or lighter than the other? Bigger or smaller? Or are things balanced equally? Is there a particular texture or color or pulsation that you sense anywhere in your torso?

Do you have a sense of your backbone leaning against the chair? Do you feel more up in your neck area or lower down in your sacrum? Or does your energy feel the same throughout?

Allow yourself to move gently, if you wish, in order to feel more in your spine. Does your spine feel solid and steady, or is there less sensation here? Notice how connected you feel to the bones of your spine right now. No judgment.

Simply noticing.

[Pause]

Now allow your attention to drop down to your pelvis, to your connection to the chair you're sitting on. What is the sensation of your sitting bones contacting the chair? Is one side resting more fully than the other, or are they balanced equally?

Notice the sensation in your upper legs, of your thighs resting on the chair. Do they feel connected to your body? Can you sense the bones of your thighs?

And your knees? Do they feel different from each other or the same? Stiff or flexible? Do you sense any particular colors or textures?

How about your calves? What do they feel like? Do you have a sense of them being a long way from your head and torso, or do they feel connected and strong? Do they feel alike, or is one more relaxed than the other? Or denser than the other?

How do your feet feel? Notice if the sensations are different or the same for both feet. What do your toes feel like? Do you feel your heels as keenly as you feel the arches and balls of your feet? Are both feet resting easily and fully on the floor, or does one feel more connected than the other? Simply noticing.

Now take a moment to scan through your entire system again, taking another overall, broad-brush look at your internal landscape, as you did when you began. As your awareness deepens, what are you noticing? Are there any changes since you first scanned your body? Take note of any sensory information: colors, textures, areas of dark or lightness, symmetries or asymmetries. Being curious and simply noticing.

[Pause]

When you are done, let your awareness return to the outer world. Gently open your eyes and notice how the world around you feels now compared to when you began. And thank yourself for taking this time to deepen your internal awareness.

EXPLORATION 2

The Core Embodiment Process

Nourishing and Replenishing the Container of Your Being

Welcome to Exploration 2.

Let yourself begin by settling in. And as this process unfolds, allow yourself to naturally, effortlessly respond to the following suggestions and questions, knowing that the ideal response is whatever spontaneously shows up in your body and in your conscious awareness as we go. This exploration is the core practice of the embodiment process. The nature of your experience will naturally change and deepen with repeated practice.

Again, make yourself comfortable, with your eyes closed or partially closed and your feet resting easily and fully on the floor. And again, invite your curiosity, your openness to discovery, to lead your conscious awareness in this exploration, so you can release any expectations or judgments as you go.

Following your breath, allow your awareness to drop into your internal landscape, feeling the rise and fall of your rib cage with each inhale...and exhale...breathing normally and noticing the sensations...the temperature of the air in your nostrils, the feel of the air traveling down into your lungs, your chest rising and falling, the feeling of your backbone on the chair. Simply noticing…being curious.

Where are you more present in your body in this moment and where are you not — where is there ease and comfort or… numbness or pain? Take a sensory snapshot that gives you a beginning reference point.

Breathing comfortably, allow your awareness to drop on down through your torso. Are your sitting bones resting equally on the chair? How do your knees feel today? How do your feet feel resting on the floor? Simply notice; no judgment.

[Pause]

Now we are going to make contact with the earth, right down through the floor and into the ground, connecting with its rich and abundant energy.

Allow your attention to drop down beneath your feet, into the earth's field as though you were putting down roots of awareness, or perhaps light beams of awareness, or maybe riding a river of awareness — use whatever imagery works for you. We are mindfully, intentionally connecting to a safe external resource that is with us all the time — the earth's field.

What does the earth feel like under you? Let sensation hits come without judgment. Is it cool or warm? Is it hard-packed and rocky? Or are you moving through sand or loose soil? Give yourself permission to take in these sensation hits — this information, even if you don't know exactly where they're coming from.

Now allow your awareness to go deeper into the earth, as though there is no resistance. Traveling down your roots or light beams or flowing on your river of awareness — going as deeply as it feels comfortable for you right now.

Perhaps your roots are on their way to the core of the earth, or you may be spreading a carpet of tiny roots right on the earth's surface. Or in this moment you may just be able to feel the earth touching your feet, but may not yet be comfortable extending your awareness down into it.

Wherever you are is fine. Simply notice what sensations show up when you get curious as to what the earth feels like under you.

[Pause]

Allow yourself to notice what you can feel in this connection outside of yourself that's safe, unconditional, and supportive.

And if you are feeling any excess tension, give yourself permission to simply let it go. You can take a deep breath and exhale the tension — take a moment now to simply inhale and exhale.

Or you can allow it to flow like water, down and out into the earth.

Or you can release it through the pores of your skin, like moisture evaporating on a cool breeze. Simply allowing yourself to let go of whatever excess tension you may have, whatever you no longer need.

And now, setting the intention to receive only what is most nurturing and nourishing, starting with your attention down in your feet, invite the earth's energy field to begin to fill your body — your container — by asking yourself, "What sensation would feel most nurturing and nourishing in my feet right now?"

Then notice what sensations show up — warmth or coolness?

Do you feel a deep pulsation or maybe a hum? Be alert to all sensory cues.

Does it feel like a particular color? Perhaps a cool blue-green or a warm red-orange or some other color?

Allow your feet to gently soak up nurturing sensations — coming up through the earth and in through your skin, soaking into all your muscles, ligaments, and tendons, letting every cell fill, all the way into the very core of your bone marrow and all the way out to your skin as best you can in this moment.

Bones are like sturdy sponges, filled with many tiny air spaces. So allow your bones to soak up this nurturing, nourishing sensation as though they were sponges soaking up clean, clear water.

Your feet may feel like they are becoming longer and wider as they fill. You may notice that one foot fills more fully or a little more quickly than the other.

Or you may simply experience an increased awareness — as you intend to let your feet receive nurturing sensation, they may simply feel different.

Do your best not to judge how much or how little you may be feeling.

Let your curiosity lead the way, and simply notice what sensations show up.

Moving at a pace that works for you, invite that nourishing feeling up into your ankles. Again, allow the sensation to soak all the way into your bones and all the way out to your skin, asking your ankles what would nourish them most in this moment?

How about your shins and calves? What would feel most nurturing there? Coolness or warmth, pulsating or humming? Perhaps the sensation — the feeling — of a long, slow stretch? Allow yourself to receive whatever sensation would nourish your calves and shins right now...letting all your cells fill up and plump out — as best you can right now.

What would feel most healing and energizing in your knees? Let that sensation permeate all the nooks and crannies of your knees, soaking up this replenishing energy.

And as we go along, if there is an area that has a harder time receiving nurturing sensation, simply notice it, allow that place to receive what it can, and cradle it gently with your awareness. Then move on, always going at your own pace.

How about your thighs? Allow this nourishing sensation to soak from the bone marrow of your thighs all the way out to your skin...letting it flow from the earth up through your feet and calves and knees right into your thighs.

This is a river of nourishing sensation you are bathing in and soaking up right now.

Rounding the curve, allow a sense of safe, nurturing sensation to soak into the sturdy bones that form the pelvic bowl.

What would feel most nourishing and healing to your sitting bones, deep into your hip bones, your sacrum — that V-shaped bone at the base of your spine — the entire pelvic bowl...soaking up this nourishment like a sponge in a clear pool of water.

What would feel most nurturing and energizing in your belly? Take a nice deep breath, cradle this area with your awareness and perhaps your hands, and let it fill and relax.

You may notice the area around and under your navel as you cradle it, gently opening in its own time, perhaps filling up from the river of nurturing sensation in your legs, on into your belly, and then moving all the way back to your spine, and all the way out to your sides — all at a pace that works for you, in a manner that works for you. Letting your reproductive system, your genitals, and your digestive system soak in nourishing, energizing sensation.

Allow the other organs of your belly and midsection to receive what they need to feel energized and relaxed and full of life.

And if you notice your mind wandering for a moment, simply bring your attention back — *Oh, yes, I was taking the time to slow down and nurture myself.*

Let this flow of nourishing energy permeate your spine....Is it warm or cool? Does it feel like a particular color? Notice as each vertebra, all the way up, and the spinal cord inside the vertebral canal, soak up whatever would feel most healing and nurturing right now.

It's helpful to breathe easily and as deeply as you can during this phase because the breath moves the spine from the inside out and gives you more sensory awareness of it.

[Pause to breathe.]

Also, feeling your spine against the chair or whatever is supporting you gives you even more sensory information about your backbone.

If you find any area where there is pain, you may notice that, for a moment or two, the pain intensifies. If so, just simply allow yourself to be with it as best you can. You're not trying to change or force the pain out; you're just gently sitting with it and allowing it to receive whatever nurturing and nourishing energy it can in this moment.

And you may find that where the rest of your body wants a rosy red color, an area that's in pain may seem to want some other color, perhaps a nice cool blue, green, or a clear silver color. Allow it to soak up whatever nurturing it can.

Now, what would feel most nurturing in your chest, your lungs, and your heart? Perhaps the sense of an easy full breath... bringing fresh oxygen to your lungs and then your heart and on out to all your cells as you inhale and exhale.

[Pause to inhale and exhale.]

And what would feel most relaxing and energizing to your shoulders...your upper chest and back? I often summon the feeling of snuggling in a soft blanket. What would feel most nourishing to you here in your shoulders right now?

[Pause]

Continue to relax and receive the sensations of nourishing yourself, taking in only what is most nurturing to you right now. Often your mind doesn't know the answer when you ask internally — and yet a sensation shows up that feels relaxing or energizing or nurturing. Simply open and receive it as best you can.

And what would feel most relaxing and energizing in your arms, your upper arms, your elbows, your forearms, down into your hands? You can gently let your fingers stretch out to draw the nurturing flow down your arms into your hands and fingers.

And what would feel most nourishing to your neck and

throat? Coolness or warmth? Perhaps a sensation of spaciousness or movement? What would feel most healing and energizing here? Allow yourself to receive it as fully as you can right now.

What about your face, your jaw, your eyes? What sensation would feel most relaxing and nurturing here?

Allow that nurturing sensation to filter all the way through to the back of your head, filling and relaxing your entire brain, all the membranes and surrounding structures and bones, soaking up nourishing sensation.

Tune in to this flow of nurturing energy filling you…filling all of you…coming in from the earth under you, through your feet and legs, through your torso and neck, arms and hands, all the way up into your head, filling and nurturing you all the way up to the crown of your head…until it begins to move out the crown, showering down around you like a gentle fountain, bathing your skin and the energy field that runs through it and around it.

If your head feels a little closed at the top, like a slight sensation of pressure, gently and slowly pull up on your hair right there at the crown, or rub your head until you feel it open, allowing this river of energy to flow out, showering down around you.

So we're nearing the end of this exploration.

When you're ready, gently notice how you feel now compared to when you began. Simply notice.

You've just connected, grounding into the earth, receiving its nourishment and support. You have created a fuller, stronger energy field within yourself and bathed in it for quite a while. You have strengthened your personal boundaries, the membrane between you and the world. This allows you to connect more deeply when you choose to and to feel strong enough to say no when you need to. It gives you clarity to see yourself and the world around you and the energy to cope with whatever arises. Notice how you feel now compared to when you began. This nourishing energy is always available to you through this process and is your core access to building a strong, nurturing container for your own life's energy and pleasure.

And when you're ready, bring your awareness back from the internal to the external. Feel your feet on the floor as you open your eyes. Allow yourself to drink in your surroundings, being informed and nurtured by all you see.

And enjoy!

EXPLORATION 3

Healing the Internal Resistance to Life

Segment 1: Core Level Physical Healing

Welcome to Exploration 3.

This exploration is done in three segments. You may stop after any of the three segments or go all the way through. The first segment explores a physical place of resistance, the second segment addresses limiting beliefs and painful recurring thoughts, and the third segment is on healing relationships. They are in this order because they build on each other. You will be given the option to stop the session at the end of each segment (signaled by a ten-second silence), or you can cruise on through the entire exploration.

So make yourself comfortable, with good back support and your feet planted easily and fully on the floor, readjusting your position as needed during the process, eyes closed or slightly open. Allow your mind to glide into neutral, releasing any expectations, agendas, or judgments you may be aware of right now. As best you can, let yourself simply experience this process.

Take a couple of easy breaths, settling back into your body. Scan through your whole internal landscape, noticing all the sensations and textures, easily filling and energizing, connecting to the earth or whatever unconditional resource works best for you at this time, so that you are beginning this exploration full and energized.

[Pause]

Now, bring to your awareness the area of your body where you feel most at home, where you feel a strong sense of connection. It might be your heart or your belly. It might be your feet, or your pelvis, or your hands. It could be your backbone. Wherever you feel the strongest sense of presence, let your awareness go and rest in that place right now and feel the fullness, the strength of that place.

It will probably feel very comfortable to be there. It is easy to rest into this place.

Take a moment now to soak up a little more from the earth's field of energy, allowing nourishing sensation into this area, so that it begins to expand and spread out, perhaps pulsating with life energy.

And in this place of strength and presence, let yourself feel or see or sense a ball of healing presence or energetic healing hands, emitting energy that is loving, patient, nurturing, strong, yet soft. This place contains unconditional love for you, which you may feel as comfort or support in some way. So, if energy hands feel right for you, use that. If a ball of healing presence works best for you, work with that image.

Sense or feel or see this healing energy in whatever way you can.

Sometimes you just *know* that it's there. Even if you don't know how you know, that's fine.

Some of you will be able to vividly *see* this healing presence or your energy hands; you'll have a color, a pulsation, a texture.

Some of you will clearly *feel* this healing presence. You'll feel the warmth and strength. Simply allow yourself to have an awareness of this energy presence, in whatever way you can.

Next, ask to be shown what block or place of resistance in

your body would be best for you to work with today. Notice what pops into your conscious awareness after you've asked.

It may be a surprise to you, or it may be a familiar place, a place where you've often felt resistance or pain. You may feel a restricted sensation in this place or a sense of disconnection from the energy flow in the surrounding areas.

You may know exactly where this is, or you may need to look around a little, asking your body to show you more clearly. Sometimes there will be pain or numbness there, or maybe it's a place that resonates with a limiting or painful phrase you often hear in your head.

Perhaps you experience it as a place of trapped emotion, such as grief or rage, sadness or shame. If you discover more than one troubled area, ask to be shown which one would be best for you to work with today. Trust what your body shows you.

Feel the edges of this place. Does it have a color? Does it have a shape? Notice.... What size is it?

If it begins to feel overwhelming, let it rest back in your consciousness for a moment, and take your awareness back to your place of greatest strength and comfort, and then down to your feet, tuning up your connection to the unconditional rich energy field of the earth.

When you are ready, allow your awareness to return to that part of you where you feel most at home — and to the ball of healing presence or the energy hands that live in that area of your body where you feel most connected.

Allow this healing presence, your energy hands, to expand from your place of strength and to gently cradle the place that feels painful or disconnected or resistant — gently, with no expectations.

If your actual physical hands can hold this place easily and without straining, allow them to join your energy hands or presence in cradling this spot.

These hands are not here to change this resistant part of you — your healing presence has no agenda. It is simply loving, caring, and strong — unconditionally holding and loving the part of you that feels disconnected (perhaps feeling hurt, ashamed, or unworthy in some way).

If you are holding a physical sensation of pain, like a lump of grief in your throat, or an area of pain in your heart, or a clutch of fear in your gut, just gently cradle that place and let the pain or the grief or the fear or the shame emerge at its own pace to connect with the healing energy hands or presence.

There is no agenda. Your pain and resistance is there for some reason. And perhaps that reason is outdated. But most likely there was a valid reason when it began, and it may now be a defense you no longer need.

It's not important to understand it now. Simply hold it and love it. Loving in the *agape* definition of love — all-encompassing, unconditional love for yourself, as though you were cradling a sleeping kitten or puppy.

Just gently cradle it. You are simply there to be with that aspect of yourself. You are not *doing* anything *to it*. You're not going to throw it away. You're not going to try to make it disappear. You are simply there with it.

This can be challenging, particularly if you are holding a place of chronic pain. You may already feel more aware and connected to that painful place than you want to be, habitually feeling the edges of it and managing your day around it.

But if you can allow yourself to go deeper today, you'll find that you are not truly connected with this place. You have been holding it at bay, controlling it — in order to be able to tolerate it. So let the edges of the pain just gently be with those energy hands or that healing presence. Simply be present, connecting with the pain, with the grief, with the sadness, whatever it is.

And if you start to feel overwhelmed by the emotion or the

pain, let it take a backseat for a moment and return to feeling your feet on the ground, feeling the energy flowing up through your body, backing up the support of your healing energy hands or presence, restoring the strong, safe container around the process, around this issue that's going on.

And when you're ready, return to gently cradling it, noticing what happens. Noticing what happens as you hold it. No expectations. Often, this is the hardest part. Your mind may have a different agenda that sounds like this:

Oh, but I want to get rid of it.

Oh, but I'm so tired of this pain.

Oh, I hate this feeling.

Whatever the words are, let them go on by. Let the judgment go and allow yourself to simply be there, connecting more and more with that part as best you can in this moment.

Accepting what is without letting it drive your bus or take over your existence. Reminding yourself that this place of pain or grief is not all of you; it is only a part of you.

You also have your feet under you. You have your energy flowing and surrounding this area. You have this strong energy presence holding and loving this part of you as best you can at this point. As best you can.

And as things begin to soften and change, remind yourself to simply be with this place — don't slip into doing something with it.

Remember the unconditional love that you're offering to this part of you. Consciously, we do not want this pain or emotion, but these are deep, long-held patterns that require our patience and compassion to transform and integrate.

In my experience, one of the most effective ways to have pain change in a permanent way is to learn how to find a way to release it from its tightened-down state, unlocking it from its prison. To do this you need to become one with it, to connect with it deeply, so that it can be free to heal.

So check in again.

How is it feeling now?

What's happening?

Notice as things change, as they evolve, honoring your own pace, holding that place in your awareness, cradling and loving it unconditionally, allowing whatever arises to unfold. Don't stand in the way.

If you notice the edges of your painful place starting to spread out and disperse, let it happen — widen your cradling presence, creating a larger space for it, so that it can evolve and transform when it is ready. Staying connected to it, but allowing it to heal and change at its own pace, so integration is more complete when it finally occurs.

And notice how this place feels now compared to when you began this process. Allow yourself to notice the small subtle changes as well as the big ones. Just simply being with this place with gratitude for all the healing, large and small, that may have occurred here today.

And gently let this place know that you will continue to hold it with loving presence, even though your conscious awareness may go elsewhere.

And let this part of you know that you have made a commitment to reconnect with it and that your internal healing presence, your energy hands, will stay with this place as long as is required to heal and transform and reconnect with the rest of you...until it is completely integrated, whether that process takes a few minutes or a few months or a few years. You are now committed to healing and integrating this part of you back into the whole.

Segment 2: Working with Limiting Beliefs

Now let's work with the way in which your mind and, specifically, your limiting beliefs and painful thoughts come into this process. Most of us are aware of the inner critical voice that can plague us with doubting, shaming, chiding, even insulting thoughts, often denigrating our self-worth or questioning our right to exist.

To begin, bring to mind one of your painful thoughts or limiting beliefs — perhaps the one associated with the physical place of resistance that you just held and loved, or notice any limiting or painful thought that is bothering you right now.

Notice where you feel that thought reverberating in your body.

Where does it anchor in your system?

Oftentimes a very painful thought will reverberate or be anchored in a pretty specific area, like your heart, or in a part of your body where you may have chronic pain, or a place that was traumatized at some point in the past, like your throat or belly, or anywhere, actually.

Simply notice where the connection is between the painful or limiting thought and your body. If it seems to connect to everywhere, notice where the connection seems the strongest or densest; it may be a familiar place.

Wherever the anchor of your pain or discomfort is, allow your internal healing presence, your energy hands, to come and cradle that place as we proceed, loving it as unconditionally as you can in this moment.

No agenda. Simply being present with it, holding it gently and witnessing it in the kind, unconditional way you just finished practicing.

Now, silently repeating your limiting belief or painful thought, ask yourself, "Am I sure that this limiting belief is true?"

Can you open to the possibility that this thought is not true at some level?

Really, you don't know whether it's true or not. Even though you may have a lot of data from past history to back up the fact that it might have been true at some point, you really don't know whether it is still true.

So now ask yourself, "What would it feel like if I were open to the possibility that this painful thought or limiting belief is not true? What would it feel like?"

And make this question very specific to whatever your painful thought is. For example, if the thought is "I am not good enough," you might say instead, "I'm open to the possibility that this thought of not being good enough is just not true. I'm open to the possibility that *I am good enough.*"

When you are ready, you can go a step farther and say, "I'm open to the possibility not only that am I good enough, but that who I am *is a pleasure*...is a pleasure."

Notice how that feels inside when you can say that to yourself and sit with it, believing it, if only for a moment.

Letting all internal judgments go silent.

What does it feel like in your body?

What's the sensation in the area now being cradled by those wonderful energy hands? Simply notice.

What would it feel like in your body if you could suspend that limiting belief and feel the ways in which you are a pleasure?

Allow that area to fully receive that possibility, even if it is only for a short while right now.

Allow yourself to open even more to that possibility.

[Pause]

What does that feel like? Feeling that you truly are a pleasure.

[Pause]

Can you feel any of the tightness dissipating?

[Pause]

Can you feel more ease in this place?

[Pause]

Can you feel any expansion inside as your perceptual lens expands?

[Pause]

Allow the healing process to unfold. Good.

[Pause]

This process takes positive affirmations all the way to the core of your being because you are actually feeling *in your body* — physically sensing — what it is like to open to new possibilities. This allows you to heal not just mentally, but emotionally and physically and, thus, spiritually as well.

And notice how this place feels now compared to when you began this process. Allow yourself to notice the small subtle changes as well as the big ones. Simply being with this place with gratitude for all the healing, large and small, that may have occurred here today.

And let this place you've been holding and loving — and dialoguing with — gently know that you will continue to hold it with loving presence, even though you may not have it in your conscious awareness as you go on back out into your life.

And you may want to commit to returning to this exploration tomorrow and perhaps the next day if something still remains that needs your conscious attention to bring it to completion. So take a moment and see what commitment, no matter how small, you want to make to yourself in terms of this healing process, and then commit to it for as long as it takes.

Segment 3: Working with Interpersonal Issues — Relationships

This process also works with issues that are on an interpersonal level.

Not surprisingly, stresses and problems in relationships are often the source of great internal pain and discomfort.

Right now, you might be carrying around a ball of fear or anger or shame or grief from a fight with your spouse or your teenager, with a work colleague or your best friend. When this occurs, you know that in this relationship something is just not working. The energy is not flowing between you. The connection is not there the way you want it to be.

The following segment will help you shift how you relate to this situation or relationship pattern, starting with your own reactions and moving on to finding new healing possibilities for yourself and perhaps for the other people involved.

Take a moment now to tune up your connection to the earth and make sure you are feeling full and energized.

Next, bring to mind the person, situation, or relationship pattern that feels painful or uncomfortable to you right now. As that sinks in, allow yourself to notice the underlying painful thought, the limiting phrase, the internal words that go along with this person or situation.

It might be similar to the limiting belief you just worked with or it could be something like:

"I'm just unlovable."

Or, "I am not safe."

Or, "I feel overwhelmed."

Or, "I'm being abandoned."

Or, "I believe I am bad — I am a tyrant."

When a belief like this dominates your thinking, it narrows your perceptual lens, keeping you from feeling the good connections you want to have with this person. Take a moment now and look for the words that reverberate through you to that ball of painful emotion in your body somewhere.

[Pause]

And once again, bring your internal nurturing hands or healing energy presence to that tight place in your body where your limiting belief is anchored and hold it unconditionally and lovingly as you've done in the previous explorations.

Then begin to expand your perceptual lens on this issue by saying something like, "I'm open to the possibility that this relationship could be different, that this relationship could heal

— could have pleasure in it again. I'm open to the possibility that I could be connected in a healthy way with my husband/teenager/friend/colleague."

Now, the tricky part of this is to hold that possibility, and expand your perceptual lens, without letting your left brain jump in immediately trying to problem solve and figure it all out.

Your challenge is to stay in an open feeling state, keeping your expansion and awareness in the realm of possibility, keeping it in the soft, diffuse place where the creativity to resolve the problem will begin to stir and show you the next step in a healing direction, or perhaps even the whole picture.

So you just hold the thought, "I'm open to the possibility. I have no idea what it would look like. Even if in my conscious mind I cannot imagine how this could be true, I'm open to the possibility that this relationship could heal and be a pleasure again, that it could work, that we could have a connection again around this issue or in this particular area. I don't know how, but I'm open to that possibility."

And then pay attention to what happens in your body. Feel your feet. Feel your torso. Feel your shoulders. Feel the place being cradled by your loving, powerful energy hands.

Allow it to shift and change as you feel into this new possibility. Simply cradling it, loving it, and letting go of judgments as they show up.

When you are able to open your perceptual field and you are willing, really willing, to be open to new possibilities, things are bound to unfold in some very interesting ways in your being.

From my own experience, both personally and as a teacher, many long-standing or complex issues, between couples especially, are not so quickly and easily resolved.

Sometimes I will need to hold the possibility for healing and reconnection for weeks or months, through many repetitions of this exploration, before I can really begin to feel in a clear, solid way the direction that I need to go to create that healing, because my resistance and my ego are so strongly attached to the problem.

Perhaps I don't want to admit that I've made a mistake or was wrong about something. Or I don't want to admit to myself or to my partner my part in the process that has separated us. So, although the steps in this process are pretty straightforward, it's not necessarily an easy path to take.

Consistent effort, persistence in using the process, trusting that there is an answer somewhere, and holding open the possibility are the keys here. When you add these to the kindness and gentleness of the unconditional presence you are holding for yourself, you have a winning combination.

Or if you feel particularly stuck or hopeless, the following phrase can be helpful: "I'm open to the possibility that this issue is not as it seems, that I am missing something, that there may be another way to see this — the whole truth of this issue may not yet be evident."

Sit quietly with these words and be open to new information. See what pops into your awareness. Watch your dreams. Ask to be shown the whole picture, open again, and listen for the still small voice of deeper wisdom to whisper to you.

Another effective tactic in resolving these stubborn, painful situations is to make a commitment to remember the possibility that you're holding as you go through each day, in your contact with this person or with the issues that bring up the pain or discomfort within yourself.

Make a commitment to remember it differently.

Make a commitment to be open to the possibility, to expand your perceptual lens around this particular issue, so that if there is another truth to be seen, it will show itself.

And sometimes when we are feeling stuck, we have to look in the mirror. Is a part of you fighting this process because you don't want to admit your role in it?

Can you gently hold that part of you and look it in the eyes and admit to yourself that you do have a role in this situation, and without blame or criticism, simply acknowledge it and move on to creating a solution, a new way of seeing yourself and the other person in this situation?

Sometimes as your perceptual lens expands, you are suddenly able to hear people around you telling you things that can help you see your issue in a new way — things that you weren't open to hearing before.

And then events spontaneously happen around you that show you things, that help you to see things with new eyes.

When we're present, with our eyes wide open, we learn from everything that happens in our lives, rather than just repeating the same events over and over again.

None of us want our most painful events to be repeated over and over. We often just don't see any other way. So make a commitment to be open to the possibility that you could see things in a new way.

Take a moment now and check in again with the part of you being cradled by your internal healing hands or presence. How does it feel now?

As you've considered new possibilities and expanded your perceptual lens, how has that impacted this place?

Has it started to shift and expand a little or a lot? Are you feeling the edges of some new ways to see your situation? Good. Wherever you are with this is fine.

And sometimes the most important step in resolving a tangled, seemingly intractable relationship problem is to make a commitment to set aside time to do this exploration on a regular basis, so that you have a vehicle to move your issue toward resolution, step by step, while holding yourself in a loving, powerful way.

So take a moment to commit to whatever you need to do,

no matter how small, if this issue needs more conscious airtime from you.

And let this part of you know that, although you are going to take your conscious awareness elsewhere as we finish up, you remain committed to this healing process as long as it takes, whether it takes a few minutes or a few months or a few years.

And now, bring your awareness back to your feet and feel the earth beneath you, soaking up what you need in order to end this process full, with that flow moving through you, feeling ready to bring your awareness back from the internal to the external, feeling full and juicy.

When you are ready, open your eyes and drink in your surroundings. Feel your backbone against your chair. Feel the steadiness of your body. Notice how you feel now compared to when you began.

And enjoy!

5 Your Heart
The Gift of Inspiration

The inner fire is the most important thing mankind possesses.

— EDITH SÖDERGRAN

The heart is the wellspring of our inspiration for life. The characteristic wisdom of the heart is in how it *inspires* us to live more deeply and fully and to create from our gifts. The energy of love resides throughout the entire body. It is the foundational energy upon which our creative inspirations are born.

Although the energy field of the heart has been proven to be quite powerful, in our culture today the voice of the heart is often muted or ignored altogether.[1] When our heart's intelligence isn't activated, we can easily feel confused, or we may listen only to the voice of the head telling us what we *should* do. The inspiration of our deepest heart's knowing is then lost to us.

There is a distinct feeling when we drop into our heart and let it open up. When we share from our heart, there is an authenticity and vulnerability that create a feeling of connection and intimacy if the listener is open and receptive.

There is also a distinct feeling when we are *not* connected

Heart Idioms

Here are things we say about our hearts and their characteristic wisdom or knowing:

My heart goes out to you.
Have a heart!
My heart sank!
She is hard-hearted.
Eat your heart out!
My heart was in my throat!
Can you find it in your heart?
His heart was racing.
My heart swells with pride.
I feel lighthearted.
My heart is filled with love for you.
My heart is just not in it anymore.
He gave it a half-hearted attempt.
That gives my heart pause.
From the bottom of my heart, I thank you.
That touched my heart.

to our heart. This could manifest as "coldheartedness," which might be experienced as a chill in the room or a conversation killer, and it will create a block to genuine intimacy.

Another feeling occurs when we are in our heart in an overly sympathetic manner. These kinds of interchanges often feel cloying, sometimes suffocating, and frequently invasive.

Yet another experience occurs when our heart resonates with another person's heart. A warmth in meeting, ease of connection, feeling deeply seen and heard — these are the empathetic connections that may become lifelong relationships or enduring imprints on our heart.

What is the quality of energy that our hearts generate? The heart expresses warmth, compassion, forgiveness, empathy, loving-kindness, and most of all inspiration. A full-hearted person is a happy person.

In Chinese medicine, the element of the heart is fire, and there is a distinct sensation when this element is balanced. We feel excited, creative, and "on fire" for life. The heart is the birthplace of our deepest inspirations, so when it has been suppressed or exhausted, we may have a flat, muted experience. Burnout approaches when our creative fire has gone out.

Priming the Deep Well of the Heart

The heart is the home of compassion. When I work with someone in the helping professions, especially healthcare providers, their genuine concern for others is apparent. Their warmth and caring is frequently the original inspiration that moved them toward their profession.

However, when I sit with them long enough, I often discover that they are much better at giving than receiving. The front of a caregiver's heart — the part that they radiate love from — feels warm and wide open.

However, often they have much less awareness of the back of their heart, the heart space of *self-love* and *nurturing*. I think of this as the deep well that feeds the rest of the heart. Like any well, when it is not primed and replenished, it runs dry and burnout starts to take hold. The front of the heart — the part shared with the world — needs connection to the deeper well of the heart in order to survive and thrive.

This means self-care is mandatory, not optional. The airlines truly do have it right. You *must* "put your own oxygen mask on first" before helping those in need around you. What the flight attendant doesn't say is that if you fail to care for yourself first, unconsciousness or even

He has a heart of gold.
She had a change of heart.
My heart shrinks in fear.
He has a heart of stone.
That was a cold-hearted remark.
I need to have a heart-to-heart conversation.
My heart stood still.
My heart aches for your loss.
She's a bleeding heart.
In my heart of hearts, I know what you are saying is true.
I am losing heart over this.
He is a man after my own heart!
She didn't have the heart to tell him no.
He broke my heart.
She felt so heavy-hearted.
She was so soft-hearted.

death may result. Yet many of us have been taught to ignore our own needs as we focus on caring for those around us. This is a sure recipe for disaster. Now is the time to turn this paradigm around and treat our own heart as a primary resource that is to be treasured and deeply valued.

The heart is the home of our deepest inspiration and the well of our love for life. Having respect for the wisdom of the heart and living from its rich depths is essential.

Woman on a Mission

Monique is a highly successful advertising executive with a wide circle of good friends as well as a close-knit immigrant family. She is well loved in her community for her generosity of heart and her sharp, clear mind. This combination of bigheartedness and clearheadedness has created success for her at every turn. Her issue is that as a mother and wife, a successful businesswoman and community member, she often feels stretched thin and exhausted, which she will admit in her quieter moments.

As an intelligent woman, Monique cognitively knows about the need for self-care. She knows she deserves to take care of herself. She also sees how valuable she is to the people in her life. But until she worked with me, she had never slowed down enough to actually experience the effects of her lifestyle on her deep physiology, specifically, her heart.

When our session started, I asked her to scan her internal sensations. She was drawn right into the area of her heart. She described it as "burning." I asked her whether it was a good burn, like a warm campfire, or whether it was something that was burning out of control. She told me it was the latter — and that it was burning extremely hot so that it could keep up with the pace of her life.

I asked Monique how far back in her chest she could feel the heat. She described it as being primarily in the front half of her chest. I knew how much energy and caring she generously spreads throughout the circles of her life. She is someone who gives a hug or shares her warm smile with anyone in need around her. She is a true gift to her world. I also knew the price Monique was paying for the way she operated from the front of her heart: her pervasive tiredness, which she could feel when she slowed down to listen internally.

I wanted to help Monique understand how to support her heart, so I shared with her about the nature of the back of the heart and how it is like a deep well — connecting us to an even deeper aquifer of life energy. This well is the place of self-love — not self-ishness, nor self-centeredness, but of the care and keeping of the soul. This well needs to be primed and regularly drawn from with true acts of self-love. This well is then the resource for all other acts of love we offer to the world — feeding the front of the heart and sustaining all the loving and sharing we do for those around us. In fact, when the deep heart is open, primed, and connected, the love we extend to the world has an effortless quality — and in our giving, we are touched as deeply as the receiver.

Monique got quiet as I spoke. I asked if this had anything to do with loving herself. Tears welled up as she shared about being a young child who was praised for loving others. She figured out at an early age how to put others' needs before her own, and she became very good at knowing and addressing the needs of others so that they were pleased with her. She had long ago muted that quiet, wise voice within.

I sensed that if this session went well, her empathy — her capacity to feel deeply and sense accurately what was going on in those around her — was about to return to being the asset it was meant to be.

Monique dropped her awareness back to her spine, behind her burning heart, and let herself spread out and relax there. I asked her to notice the sensations in the front of her heart as it loosened up and connected to the resource of the deep well of the back of her heart. The burning sensation diminished slowly as she explored this area.

Monique visibly relaxed as she settled back in her body — as she felt her heart, she said, "come into a friendlier relationship with the rest of my body." She was starting to feel her spine and the steadiness of her bones.

A smile came to her face as Monique described the sensations "coming in for a landing" as she rode the wave of feeling down her spine to her pelvis. We continued to explore and add to the support for the heart by playing with what it would feel like to inhabit her legs and feet as well. This went more slowly, but by the time we ended, she was feeling rooted down into the earth's rich energy field.

As I scanned her field in closing, I noticed that her heart energy had naturally flowed down her arms and into her hands, as well as up into her head without any help or suggestion from me. This made sense, as these pathways were ones she had honed from early on in her life. In Chinese medicine, the meridians of the heart connect us into our hands and fingers, as we naturally extend our arms to hug others when our hearts are full of love or in need of love.

As we wrapped up the session, Monique checked inside to ascertain what attitudes and actions would be loving to herself, so that she could keep this deep well primed and flowing to the front of her heart. She made an action plan and got agreement with her heart that she would take quiet time each day to listen to her inner landscape. She would do a short practice of the Core Embodiment Process (Exploration 2, pages 59–66), grounding and filling twice a day to help her sense better what she needed in any given moment. She was relaxed and settled inside herself as she left my office.

As I reflect on her journey now, I realize how much her process is mirrored by most people who are caring, loving individuals in our world today. We are not taught how to truly love ourselves in deep, nurturing ways. We don't realize the power of feeling into every corner in our heart. We have lost the fact that the heart needs to be honored throughout its entirety, not just the front part that we share. Taking that a step further, many caring individuals have grown into the people they are by learning to pay attention *outside* of themselves to the needs of others, often to the detriment of what is happening *inside*.

Feeding the Deep Heart Guides the Way Home

Julian is a dynamic, tall, handsome man in his early twenties. He came to me with deep exhaustion and anxiety that kept him on edge most of the time. When I first met him, I was struck by his earnest warmth and genuine caring for others. We did this session seated, although I did use touch to speed up the process as we worked.

As he sat with his eyes closed, I asked him to describe his life for me. I put my hands on the front of his chest and on his back behind his heart to better track what he was struggling with as he spoke. Julian runs a nonprofit for inner-city children living below the poverty line, and it inspires him deeply. What I felt as he talked about his mission with these children was a heart that is deeply inspired — my front hand felt lots of warmth exuding from his chest as he shared the details of this part of his life. My back hand felt almost no warmth or energy at all. It actually felt a little vacant.

I asked Julian whether he could feel a difference between the front of his chest and the back, and he immediately confirmed that he could feel the warmth coming from about halfway back out to the front. His back felt cold to him. I was encouraged that he had that level of awareness in the beginning of our first session. I knew this would probably go quickly with that level of opening awareness.

I explained that he was not alone in doing what I call "running slightly in front of himself" with all his inspiring activities. I felt him relax a bit when he realized that this was simply an energy habit, not a character flaw.

It is an epidemic in our culture today to adopt the energy habit of running slightly out in front of ourselves, trying to keep up with all that life offers or demands of us. However, the first problem that arises is that we lose the sense of the back of our body when we chronically live from this forward-leaning energy habit.

As I was writing this book, which deeply inspired me, I also caught my inner body awareness sliding forward out of my back, as I concentrated on the words appearing on my computer screen in front of me. So many things pull us forward in the world today, and it is so important to remember to rest back and enjoy yourself on a regular basis.

I often see people in my practice with anxiety as a result of abandoning their inner navigational system by running in front of themselves, constantly checking for safety on different levels. For some, it is physical safety. For others, it might be emotional safety, financial safety, or any kind of preoccupation with the future. The squirrel in the cage of the mind, running endlessly on the wheel of worry, is fed when you do not have access to the present moment of sensation in the exquisite navigational system of your body, which leaves only future possibilities or past experiences to go on.

I asked Julian to let his focus expand from the front to his back, where my hand cradled his spine behind his heart. Slowly, he was able to sink in. About halfway there, it stopped. I asked him what he was thinking.

"If I do not keep my awareness on red alert for safety, I will fall prey to untrustworthy people. I have to keep my awareness constantly scanning out there in front of me...." Julian trailed off, realizing what he was saying. I let him know that I would be introducing him to a better danger/safety detector in a few minutes.

Again, I felt him relax another level, and both of us could feel warmth arriving in my hand on his spine. A slow smile came to his face.

"This feels really nice — and quiet, restful, and peaceful. If I could live from here, I bet I would not feel so exhausted all the time!" A smile came to my face this time.

Now that warmth was extending from front to back fully, we could start exploring the sensations of his gut instincts — that danger/safety knowing. He easily breathed his way down his spine and into his gut. It felt easy and full. I brought his awareness to the connection between his heart and his gut. He could feel that easily as well.

Next I asked him to think of a situation where he had made a decision that he regretted. He immediately thought of a recent issue where he had felt things were off, but he had let his mental faculties overrule his gut knowing. On paper, the situation looked perfect. In real time, it was a mismatch that had made his life miserable for a month. I asked him to notice that his gut had signaled him without him constantly scanning the horizon and exhausting himself. He grinned when he realized that.

Next I asked him to think of something that he had done that was a wonderful success. He immediately brought to mind a wonderful and slightly wacky idea he had jumped into and brought to fruition easily. I asked him how *that* felt. I could feel the warmth flood his gut with "this is right for you" signals, even as his heart was feeling deeply inspired by it all. He was grinning from ear to ear remembering the whole event and how right it had felt, despite all the facts surrounding the issue. This told me he had a good relationship going between his heart and his gut. On top of that, his mental faculties had joined with his gut and his heart to strategize how to make it all work so easily. It was just *fun*!

I completed the session by walking him through the Core Embodiment Process. I showed him how to ground and fill up the rest of the container of his body by allowing a flow of energy to come in from the earth beneath him, flowing up his legs to join and support his gut, heart, and mind. When we were done, he felt relaxed, solid, and present. What a gift he will bring to the world from here!

Resilience and an Open Heart

"I am seriously wondering whether my husband and I will make it," Lila said to me during our session. "At times, I think he's really selfish and has no idea the impact of his behavior on me. I often feel vulnerable and anxious." Lila's calm demeanor and intelligent gaze belied her inner turmoil.

I asked what her husband had done to cause so much angst, and Lila replied that her husband had had three motorcycle accidents in the last three years, which had left her fried. In the last accident, he was so seriously injured that it was touch-and-go as to whether he would emerge intact. Though he had recovered fully, it took quite a while for him to do so.

I asked if, by saying he was "selfish," Lila meant that he continued to ride.

"No, he has agreed to give it up," she replied.

I asked what reassurance Lila needed from her husband. She said, "I don't know. I just feel *so* anxious all the time." At that point, we went to the treatment table so I could put hands on her to better support whatever needed to unfold.

I was immediately drawn to her heart, so I put my hands on the front and back of it. I asked her to allow her awareness to come into the space between my hands. I registered a sense of shock and frozenness that was not readily apparent on the surface. Lila was a vibrant, beautiful woman in the prime of her life. Before this series of events she was at the top of her game, both successful and highly esteemed in her professional world. With her husband's latest accident, and her weeks at his bedside, she had to put much on hold, and that suspension was also adding to her anxious and ungrounded feelings.

Ever since, Lila had been walking on eggshells, constantly on alert for what was going to happen next. This is the typical response of a system still in shock. It loses its resilience, its ability to bounce back after the adversity or trauma has passed.

I asked Lila how her heart felt to her. She said it felt fortressed and hard, as though protecting itself. I gently let her know that was normal for someone who had been through what she had been through, almost losing a loved one. I explained that the repeated shocks to her heart had caused it to tighten down to the place that felt protected, but there was no resilience left — no capacity to roll with whatever came next. She was basically hypervigilant and running on adrenaline.

"Has anyone held your heart like this since the last accident?" I asked. She said she had plenty of other kinds of support, but no one had held her heart. She was the one supporting everyone else, while trying to keep the pieces of her high-powered professional life together.

"And how does your heart feel, being held in this caring way, with no agenda and no time pressure?" I continued. Lila said my hands felt very warm, safe, and comforting. I could feel the hardness starting to soften between my hands.

Directing my next question to her heart, I asked what it needed from here. Her immediate answer was "peace." I asked Lila what *peace* meant to her heart, and she replied that it was a sense of quietness and stillness, rather than the agitation she had been living with for the last few years.

Then she said, "Freedom." I immediately thought of what

she'd first told me, that she was wondering if she and her husband would be strong enough to stay together.

When I asked what she meant, Lila said, "Freedom from this anxiety I live with constantly." Her response indicated to me that she was ready to drop a layer deeper. Her anxiety was no longer being projected onto her husband as the causal factor.

As I continued to hold her heart, I could feel the achy quality leaving her chest as it relaxed to deeper and deeper levels over the next five minutes. She shared that she could feel from the front all the way to the back, and it was one continuous flow of warmth.

Lila was concerned that she didn't know how to feel safe if part of her wasn't vigilant all the time. I asked her how she was feeling in that moment. She noted that she was not anxious anymore. I helped her connect her heart and her gut instincts so she would be signaled if something was truly wrong.

Lila realized that with her adrenaline running all the time, everything looked like a potential danger, which caused her more worry and stress. I pointed out that the gut would signal her if something in the current moment was dangerous in her environment.

I asked Lila how she was feeling about her husband. A slow smile came to her face. Her resilience had returned. Her heart was relaxed and full once more.

When I spoke to her the following week, she shared that her heart continued to feel full and that her anxiety was significantly lower. In fact, it had become negligible in her life.

Loving Halfheartedly

When Marcus, an attractive, dark-haired thirty-year-old, first came to my office, I could not quite put my finger on why I had trouble connecting with him. It was as though a glass shield existed between Marcus and the rest of the world. Superficial witty exchanges took place, but nothing of depth. When his pain surfaced on my treatment table, I was able to clearly see the pattern and consequences of loving "halfheartedly."

As my first session with Marcus began, I cradled his chest between my hands, and we both took our awareness into the area of his heart. He reported that it felt knotted up and small — maybe half its original size. When we engaged with his "half-a-heart," he suddenly remembered experiencing a deep loss in his life when he was seventeen. In a matter-of-fact voice, Marcus told me that he had ended his first deep love relationship when his girlfriend had to return to Oregon. He reported that "the breakup was inevitable, and there was nothing that could have been done to alter the outcome." His emotionless sharing indicated to me that he was speaking from his head rather than feeling the message his heart was trying to convey.

I asked Marcus what part of himself he was speaking from. He was silent for a moment and then realized his awareness had left his heart and was reporting in from his head. I gently asked him to drop back to his chest area and answer from there.

Within minutes, tears were streaming down his face. As he felt safe enough to share, he described how special she had been to him. Slowly, his heart unfurled from its tight ball, letting go of the grief of that loss. Marcus was startled and shocked by the intensity of his feelings. He had no idea how much he was carrying there. His logical mind said, "After all, it was just a young love, one that we knew from the beginning was going to end because she was visiting family for the summer."

Under my hands, his chest felt warmer and warmer as layer after layer of grief and sadness rolled out. To our amazement, after his heart expanded to its normal size, it kept right on going until Marcus had the feeling that it was filling his whole body. He was astonished by how different and real everything felt. The glass shield was gone, and the fullness of life had returned to him.

All his senses were reawakened, fine-tuned, and receiving exqui-
sitely well. His face was lit up with joy.

I met up with Marcus again recently. We spoke in depth
about that transformational session. His presence now has an authenticity to it. As we shared time together, I felt a deep, easy
connection. What a difference having his whole heart is making
to Marcus's experience of the richness and fullness in his life.

A Sense of Belonging

Caroline struggled for years with dissociation and a sense of not
feeling safe. In our early sessions together, we ascertained that these
limiting beliefs originated from early childhood sexual abuse. For
years she lived in an almost perpetual state of hypervigilance, on
red alert, tracking all the people around her. This skill made her
keenly sensitive to others' needs, but she was unable to know or
be with her own needs and comfort.

On top of that, Caroline's husband was emotionally unavail-
able and traveled most of the time, which furthered her sense of
aloneness in the world. She only felt truly at ease out in nature
with her dog. Yet she longed to feel at home — that easy sense of
belonging that she knew others had but that she lacked.

For several years, Caroline has worked with me, tenaciously
fighting her way back to reinhabiting her body with all of its sensations. Initially, my role as her facilitator was simply to help her
notice the threshold where she would begin to dissociate so she
could choose to stay present when she was ready to do so. After
months of her moving back into her torso and her pelvis, she was
finally ready to focus on her heart.

Caroline started this session by announcing that despite
all our work, and all that she had done, she still found herself
plagued by a sense of not belonging, no matter where she went,
no matter how friendly the people, no matter how hard she struggled to recognize her limiting beliefs and neutralize them. On top

of that, her beloved dog, Muffin, was dying, and that impending loss felt excruciatingly painful to contemplate.

"It hurts too badly to stay with this dying process — I need it to just be over," she said. I could tell she was feeling guilty even as those words tumbled out of her mouth.

I didn't know how Muffin's dying and her bigger life issue of feeling a sense of belonging were tied together, but it felt right to continue.

"So, Caroline, exactly which part of your heart hurts the most with the pain of Muffin's dying?" I asked.

She said the front part — it was full of searing pain that felt achy around the edges. We sat with that sensation for a moment and honored how special Muffin was for her. I asked her how it felt if she let her attention drop back behind the searing pain, into the area deep in her chest along the front of the spine.

Caroline got very quiet, and then she told me it was all very dark and very peaceful. Her love for her dog was alive and well in this part of her heart. She found no fear of loss here. In her mind's eye, she could see Muffin curled up on her lap sleeping peacefully.

As the minutes passed, Caroline realized this area, her deeper heart space, felt large, dark, and empty like a huge cave. She found it a bit unsettling to be alone in the dark with all that empty space. I asked her if anybody else was there. She replied that there were only echoes when she called out.

We sat together for several more minutes, and then Caroline noticed there were whispers all around her in the dark. Not scary whispers but comforting somehow. Initially, she could not tell what was being said, and then she started to weep softly. She told me, "They are welcoming me home. They are whispering things like, *There you are. You have come back!*"

I asked her how it felt to hear those words. As she continued weeping, she said, "Comforting — it feels comforting, like I have found where I belong, where I fit in." These were tears of joy and relief, and I could feel her relax.

Caroline said the gentle whisperings told her, *You can stop searching now.* As she experienced this place within her heart, she felt the nearly constant grip of the knot in her stomach dissolving.

She finished her session by weaving together the front and back of her heart, thus integrating this place into the totality of who she is.

Caroline found her sense of belonging in the safest of all places, deep in her own heart.

For Your Heart Only

"Falling head over heels in love with someone who is not right for me seems to be the story of my life," said Bella, a gorgeous, vibrant, twentysomething who loves with all her heart. Unfortunately, she would forget to include the inner wisdom of the rest of her body.

Bella's dilemma was apparent as I listened to the account of her latest in a string of similar love relationships.

"When I fall in love, my heart gives me a big yes — however, it is not unusual for there to be whispers of advice from elsewhere in my body suggesting that I put the brakes on, to wait and see. To be honest, I rarely, if ever, wait. Then, after diving in too soon and living with the consequences, I walk around feeling guilty for betraying myself because I did not listen to the rest of me about the rightness or wrongness of the relationship."

Bella continued, "Honestly, I don't even know if I really 'love' my latest guy because of the disconnection between my heart and the rest of me. I often end up feeling heartbroken because he wanders away or does not reciprocate to the depth that I am extending to him. Then there is the confusion inside after we have a particularly potent night together, and I feel like I'm having a drug withdrawal. He does not understand that at all, and even I feel a little crazy to feel this way."

We talked at length about her lonely brokenheartedness. Bella is a striking beauty, intelligent, and kind — a wonderful combination, but not where her own heart is concerned. I helped her explore what it would feel like to get her heart deeply connected to her gut and head. Her connections were tentative at best and easily ignored in a rush of passion.

As I showed her how to make this connection more palpable within her inner landscape, she visibly relaxed and had a more solid feeling within herself. She was becoming her own best friend.

After several years, now twenty-nine years old, Bella is in a healthy, passionate relationship — with her inner knowing guiding her choices moment to moment. In her words from a recent conversation, "I took much longer to set the foundation for this relationship. But he felt the specialness of it as well, so he was totally onboard with the pace of how it all unfolded."

The heart is meant to be held and *supported* by the lower half of the body, not betrayed by it. Yet when that pelvis/gut/heart connection is not there, the heart is often disappointed, if not broken.

In closing, there is much wonderful research about the power and intelligence of the heart and its integral relationships with all the other systems of the body, most notably the heart-to-brain and heart-to-immune-system connections.

These stories are a small sampling from the thousands I could have chosen to make the point about the heart, its characteristic wisdom, and its metaphoric anatomy, which can make all the difference in the world to our quality of life, to our sense of deep inspiration, and to whether we are thriving or burning out.

My hope is that you see some similarities in these stories with yourself and those around you. May the learning inform and deepen your embodiment in this important wisdom area of who you are as a human being.

To explore the wisdom of your heart, practice this chapter's exploration. To download the audio, go to www.healing-fromthecore.com, click on the Reclaiming Your Body Download link, and enter the password *presence*.

EXPLORATION

The Wisdom of the Heart Exploration

Feel free to do Explorations 1 (pages 55–59) and 2 (pages 59–66) prior to this exploration for a deeper experience. Also remember that Exploration 3 (pages 66–79) is designed to be used whenever you hit a roadblock or some kind of resistance in your Core Embodiment Process — so if, as you are exploring each of the different wisdom areas, you uncover some resistance, that would be an indicator to use Exploration 3 (but certainly not to give up and tell yourself the process simply does not work or does not work for you).

Inner Awareness

Begin by simply taking a baseline of your inner awareness, without trying to change anything. To do this, allow your feet to rest fully on the floor, eyes closed or semiclosed. As you settle in, following your breath, be curious about the temperature of the air as it enters your nostrils and fills your lungs.

Notice the rise and fall of your chest and back as you breathe normally.

Heart Awareness

Next, allow your awareness to travel to the area of your heart, dropping your attention inside, as deeply as is comfortable at this time.

What sensations show up here?

Does it feel warm or cool?

Does it feel like a particular color?

Is there a hum or a pulse?

The heart is well known as the home of our caring, compassion, and love. Travel to an even more profound level, and the heart is the wisdom keeper of our deepest inspirations, keeping our inner fire burning.

What is it that inspires you most in your life right now? What lights up your days and energizes you? Feel where it resides in your heart. What is the sensation of it? What images arise?

You might be inspired by a project you're involved with, or something in your own healing process, or raising a family, or creating something new and exciting.

Whatever it is, allow yourself to notice what it feels like in your heart as you breathe into and acknowledge this inspiration in your life right now.

When you are ready, allow this energy of inspiration and love to rest deeply into the back area of your heart, filling and priming the well of your deep heart. Loving and honoring who you are right now in this moment.

To embody more fully here, breathing in, feel the sensation of your backbone behind your heart leaning on whatever is supporting it right now.

[Pause]

Notice the movement sensations here along your spine as you breathe an easy deep breath.

You may want to wake up your spine here behind your heart further up by rolling forward or arching back — stretching it all out in both directions — whatever helps you expand your sensation awareness in this area of the back of your heart. Yoga is great for this. Take a moment now and allow your spine to wake up and support your deep heart.

[Pause]

Check now to make sure your back support is good, and adjust if needed to *rest back*, allowing your deep heart to be fully supported by your spine.

[Pause]

As you breathe, allow your awareness to drop down your spine and into your torso under your heart area...and on down with each breath into your belly, your sitting bones...and on down your legs, into your feet...and on through to that safe, rich, unconditional resource beneath us — the earth.

[Pause]

And having made this connection, breathe in whatever sensation would nourish you best in this moment — simply noticing the temperature, color, texture of it and welcoming it into your feet...your legs...your torso...forming a cushion of support for your heart...a steady connection of energy between the earth and your heart.

Your heart is being cradled by this rich energy source all the time when you are fully embodied and connected to the resources around you. Allow your awareness to expand to include this experience, as fully as you can in this moment.

When you are ready, let your heart receive whatever it needs and wants in this moment from this rich flow of energy — soaking it in effortlessly, filling from the deepest parts all the way to the surface — every curve and connector physically...emotionally...spiritually.

[Pause]

And as it fills and fills, allow this energy of love and inspiration to expand on out into the rest of your chest...and from there, down your arms and into your fingers.

All the acupuncture meridians of the heart reach into the fingers. This is how we transmit physically what is in our hearts, by hugging someone or reaching out and touching them. As your hands and arms fill...let them reconnect back into your heart, by holding and cradling your own heart, completing the circuit.

[Pause]

Next, allow your heart's flow to expand up into your throat and neck...awakening and nourishing your true voice as your throat softens and relaxes.

[Pause]

And to complete our journey here, allow this river of nourishing sensation to connect up into your head, your face, your brain...awakening all the circuitry here for an integrated heart-brain intelligence — a connection that is so fundamental to deeper consciousness.

[Pause]

As your cranium fills and overflows, allow the area of your crown to open, connecting you to the heavens and completing this wonderful journey.

And enjoy!

6 Your Gut

The Gift of Instinctual Knowing

Trust instinct to the end, even though you can give no reason.

— RALPH WALDO EMERSON

As you know from my game-changing story in chapter 1, about the attack that almost led to my demise, my gut knowing is what inspired this whole journey home to myself.

I have taught about it for years and watched many people learn to relax and enjoy life a whole lot more once they understand that their gut is always keeping tabs on what is happening inside and outside of themselves.

The good news is this means the worrying mind can take a vacation — the gut is a lot more accurate and can instantly let us know when something is really right and when something is really off.

The key is learning to read the signals that the gut uses. These signals are unique to each person. There are general categories — some people have a *visual* image flash through their mind, some have an actual *physical sensation* of calm or uneasiness, some *hear* a warning or a reassuring sound or voice in their head, and some have a *thought* such as, *Get up and move away from that doorway.*

Some people experience a combination of signals or have their own unique way of sensing their gut knowing.

In my thirty years of asking people about their gut knowing, I have heard thousands of stories about how a disaster was averted, or an unexpected and wonderful experience happened, because people listened to the wisdom of their gut.

Feeling into your gut knowing consistently is both easy and difficult. However, once you learn how to live from your gut, you will navigate through your life with greater grace and ease.

Why Is Gut Knowing Both So Easy and So Hard?

Most of us have had at least one life experience when our gut hunch was completely accurate. It told us something was either "spot on" or "definitely off" about a person or event, and this knowing served us well.[1] When this happens enough times, we come to trust it. We may not yet understand the physiological mechanism behind this kind of knowing, but most people have felt it demonstrated in their lives.

One explanation might be recent research on the enteric nervous system, which functions like a literal "gut brain." This part of our anatomy guides our immune system, and it also contributes to the optimum functioning of our actual brain (the one in our head) and the rest of our systems.[2] This research has firmly established that we all have gut intelligence.

If that's true, then why is accessing or trusting our gut knowing sometimes so hard? There are several common or probable reasons. One is that we often second-guess ourselves. Our rational mind may disagree with our gut brain, and we listen to our mind instead. Another is when we worry about the past or future, and this obscures our present-moment awareness so that we don't clearly hear our gut's message. And a third major reason is when we have unresolved trauma memories. The body can store those memories, walling them off to minimize their effect on the system, which allows normal daily functioning to continue. If the area that is walled off is in the gut, then the navigational functioning and clarity of that area can be diminished or impaired (as in Dr. Upledger's energy cyst model, mentioned in chapter 2).

A Traumatized Gut

I learned about the impact of trauma memories on the gut thirty years ago, while working with my first severe childhood trauma survivor. As we worked together to heal her past trauma, I was saddened to hear her tell me that she had suffered a new trauma. One night the previous week, someone mugged her in a dark parking lot coming out of her psychotherapist's office.

As she told me her story, I realized she was so frozen and compartmentalized from her childhood trauma that she had been oblivious to the danger in that parking lot. Her navigational system — her gut knowing — was not up and running for her safety and well-being that night.

Please understand, I did not blame her. She simply did not have access to what she needed in order to potentially

Gut Idioms

I had a gut feeling that would happen.

My gut reaction was to act.

Go with your gut.

Her gut response was no, even though it made no sense.

He just couldn't stomach it.

It was gut-wrenching.

Her gut said yes, even without the facts.

It was a punch in the gut.

I had butterflies in my belly.

Trust your gut.

Follow your gut.

His stomach dropped when he heard the news.

The rejection gutted me.

I hear my thoughts but I feel my gut.

Her stomach was tied in knots.

I felt intestinal certainty.

He has intestinal fortitude.

Failing the course was a gut check.

avoid that dangerous situation. Past trauma can lock us out of clear signals from the gut.

Here is another story that illustrates how clearing old trauma can allow greater trust of one's gut knowing.

Katherine's husband, Jonathan, was in the early stages of dementia, but he was understandably reluctant to give up responsibilities he was still capable of handling. The problem for Katherine, as his primary caregiver, was knowing what these were. She needed an accurate intuition more than logic to navigate, for instance, when he was clear enough to pay the bills or when he needed her help. For caregivers everywhere, this may sound like a familiar dance.

Katherine recounted how Jonathan had recently called her into his office for help with logging on to the computer. After she showed him what to do, he waved her away, assuring her he had it from there. Yet something inside guided her to stay. The reason became clear moments later. As Jonathan opened bills, they discovered an overdue insurance bill threatening cancellation of their homeowner's policy.

Katherine's chest clutched as shock waves ran through her entire body. She became so agitated she needed to leave the room. She knew this reaction was not about Jonathan or the bill, but it related to something older and deeper. This frozen, panic response to sudden change was one she had been plagued by her whole life, but without completely understanding it. Katherine recognized that this response, if it continued, would exhaust her ability to go the distance with her beloved husband and the ups and downs of progressing dementia.

I asked her to recall the entire scene with her husband, moment by moment. As she got to the place where the panicky feeling hit, I felt her freeze up inside. On top of that, she seemed not in the present moment.

I asked her, "How old do you feel right now, Katherine?"

She responded, "Five years old. I'm standing in the living room of my childhood home, feeling paralyzed with fear."

Some unexpected financial news had placed her family in shock. Being five years old, Katherine did not know the details — but the feeling response was palpable. Katherine, as a young child with no solid boundaries yet, absorbed the panic and overwhelmed emotions of her family. She felt the enormity of the situation and froze, unable to move — and this was the same feeling she had upon seeing the bold red lettering of the overdue bill fifty years later.

To process this unresolved trauma, we returned together to that moment in time with her family and offered "little" Katherine the solace and help she needed. Her body relaxed in layers, melting and releasing the frozen, overwhelmed parts.

Then we reviewed her current situation with Jonathan. In doing so, a whole new perspective emerged. Now freed from the trauma of the past, Katherine saw how her gut had reliably and accurately guided her to stay in the room with Jonathan — not leaving him alone to pay the bills that day. Her gut knew something needed her attention.

As she thanked her inner knowing, she felt her whole system relax. It was like discovering a vital and trustworthy inner partner and friend.

As we went deeper, Katherine realized how accurately her gut wisdom had been tracking how Jonathan was doing on any given day. She was flooded with memories of recent times when it had signaled important actions to take to avert problems.

The only barrier was her outdated panic response related to her old childhood memory. As she released this trauma response from her tissues, her gut was now completely unimpeded and free to signal without the old interference.

When Katherine consciously acknowledged the reliability of her gut's inner knowing and guidance, she felt a surge of well-being and confidence to navigate the future. She felt like she was shaking hands with her new partner — her gut — and promising to trust and pay attention to the signals it sends.

Without the panic and sense of overwhelm from her past trauma, Katherine looked forward to having more energy to keep herself resilient and enjoying life, even as her husband's dementia progressed. In addition, her gut would help guide her in maintaining her own self-care regime, which would keep her energy reservoir as full as possible for the coming years as she cared for her husband.

Second-Guessing Leads Us Astray

Another barrier to gut knowing is our tendency to overthink or second-guess ourselves.

Most of us think *way* too much! Western civilization encourages and honors our linear, rational minds more than our intuitive, primal gut knowing. If, as I mention above, it's common for people to experience their gut knowing at least once, that means second-guessing it is equally common. As I write in chapter 2, I know numerous brilliant people who talk themselves out of their gut knowing and drive themselves crazy by overthinking constantly.

So I want to raise a slightly different issue. Once we learn to experience and trust this kind of gut knowing, we can come to rely too heavily on an initial intuitive hit. As time goes on, we may get new information from our gut, but we ignore it and go astray because we think the issue is already decided. In other words, we value our gut knowing, but we overthink it and stop listening, and this gets us into trouble.

For instance, years ago, my old friends Janice and Bob were visiting a place they had never been, and they fell in love with it. They both agreed that it just felt right for them to live there. They went home with stars in their eyes and made plans to sell everything and move to their dream place. But was it actually a dream come true? Or might it become a nightmare? It would depend on how closely they *continued* to listen to their insides.

What can happen — and I have seen this many times with only slight variations — is that someone will feel the "rightness" of the present moment and then take action on that "right feeling." They go into their heads (leaving their gut behind) and quickly start making plans and taking action. Yet their gut sense continues to signal to them, moment to moment, with contradictory information or cautionary warnings, which they ignore.

Often, if we can stay with our present-moment gut wisdom, this signaling may say something like, "This does feel wonderful, but take it slowly." Or, "This place is great, but check the work situation: Does your license transfer easily or will you spend months or years jumping through hoops just to make an income sufficient to support yourself?" Or, "This is an excellent place to nurture yourself on vacation, but not to live permanently."

In Janice and Bob's case, they did find their dream home — complete with a garden and animals they had always wanted — and moved across the country. But they found that making a living in this new environment was much more difficult than anticipated. They had both been extremely successful professionally in their home state. Within a year, Janice decided to fly back to her private practice ten days per month in order to be able to financially afford their new life. Over the years, the stress took a toll on Janice's health, and when we last spoke, she was struggling with a chronic, stress-related health issue, leaving me wondering whether this dream was worth it in the end.

Negative Worrying Thoughts and Present-Moment Sensation

A repetitive negative thought is what we call *worry*. It is recognized by a charged sensation of some kind — an emotional reaction, the physical feeling of a hot button or pain. It may cause you to suddenly freeze or go numb when you were feeling fine only moments before. Or it may feel like a trigger has been pulled, causing your nervous system to go into its classic fight-flight-freeze response. You may find yourself trying to control this response, explain it away, or blame it on someone else. Most of all, it feels so potent that many people don't recognize its origin as coming from outside of themselves.

Often, worry runs through our mind over and over like a broken record. It may be a recording of an event from your past, which is similar to a current event. It may be a thought projection into the future based on past events. It may even be an old negative message about yourself or the world, one that keeps showing up and driving you onward. This is what happened with Tony, the nurse practitioner from chapter 3, who made choices based on his past that resulted in a devastating lack of self-care and eventually a heart attack.

Most importantly, how can we differentiate between that endless grind of negative thoughts that most of us hear inside our heads and a true gut knowing? They both can potentially cause unpleasant sensations throughout the body.

Quite simply, the gut's wisdom comes from present-moment sensations that inform us of what is happening inside or outside of ourselves. It is most often a quiet event, with very little charge to it. It is simply a statement of fact. It may reveal itself as a pleasant or not-so-pleasant sensation. It is informing you about what is going on moment to moment and whether it is right for you or off the mark.

I have studied this concept for decades and witnessed thousands of situations in my classes and practice that corroborate it. Much of my work is facilitating an inner process that helps people discern the difference between the quiet, gut knowing about the present moment and the worried, charged feeling that comes up when we remember something old, project into the future, or simply get stuck in our heads, overthinking a situation.

An Integrated Gut

With this in mind, I always advocate for what I call an *integrated gut*. I have also heard it called an "educated gut." Essentially, it means that the gut knowing is in conversation with, or integrated with, all of the other parts of your whole system — such as the heart's inspiration, the clarity of your bone-deep knowing, the capacity of your feet and legs to metabolize that knowing, and your brain's capacity to integrate and make sense of all the information coming from these wisdom areas.[3]

What most people call *intuition* is what occurs when you have an integrated gut — one that is connected to your entire system, body, mind, and spirit. When this occurs, internal wisdom-knowing abounds. Answers come when they are needed, and sometimes not a moment before.

Consider falling in love. It feels so right in the moment, but it can have heartbreaking effects if the gut, feet and legs, bones, and the rest of your system are not included. Bella (from chapter 5) continually fell in love and got her dreams crushed because she was leaving her integrated gut totally out of the equation. Once she included it, her decisions rapidly got much wiser. An integrated gut — be sure to always include it in any major decision. Don't leave home without it.

Gut wisdom shows up best when we are not thinking — such as when we are just drifting in or out of sleep or taking a leisurely walk with awareness of our natural surroundings. When we allow ourselves to move beyond our thoughts, limiting beliefs, and the expectations of other people, the gut's wisdom shines.

If, on the other hand, we fiercely hang on to a certain belief about a situation — believing it is wonderful, necessary, or the best that it can be — we often cannot hear or feel the signals telling us the situation is not supporting our health and well-being. In this case, we are no longer in the present moment. We are caught up in our head and held captive by an expectation or a limiting belief.

Years ago I worked with a woman, Julie, who desperately wanted a second child and was determined to conceive. There was no arguing with her because she "knew" best and was locked in on her mental vision of the future. It was a noble one. She herself was one of eight children, and she said, "I want my daughter to have a sibling and not grow up a lonely only child."

In our work together, I felt Julie's body was not in agreement with her mental vision. I gently held space for her to come to this knowing herself, but she was unable to get the message from her gut due to her blindingly strong desire to conceive again.

In a case like this, I know it is better to remain silent and allow the person to come to their own truth in their own time. That time came fairly quickly for her.

As it turned out, Julie *did not* conceive, and her marriage broke up shortly thereafter due to her unfaithful husband.

Julie was essentially caught in the future, with no grounding in the present. This kept her locked out of the present-moment information that this expectation was not right for her.

Of course, sometimes we try to access our gut knowing to make a decision, but we cannot seem to get an answer. In times like these, I might begin to question whether my gut wisdom is still operating. However, I have learned to simply wait. When an answer does not come, or remains foggy, it means that it's probably premature to make a decision. I need to rest back and wait for the answer to show up, to sleep and dream on it. Take a long walk and forget about it. It means that I need to stay present in the moment and not go running out into the future, trying to make the decision logically when that is not what is called for. *Living*

in the present moment of sensation is the best guide for accessing your
gut wisdom.

Practice Listening to Your Gut Wisdom

Think about a situation you are puzzling over — perhaps you
are trying to make a choice between more than one option. This
could relate to your job, a relationship, or a move you are considering.

All decisions have at least two options — option one is "don't
change," and option two is "try something else." Many times,
there is more than one something else. Whatever the case, the
internal listening process is basically the same.

Find a quiet place where you will not be disturbed. Close
or partially close your eyes. Allow yourself to drop your awareness into the area of your gut. Notice what baseline sensations
are there when your mind is clear and not contemplating either
option. Simply rest in the present moment. Does your gut feel
relaxed or tense?

A sense of excess tension might be your baseline if you have
unresolved trauma locked here. Recognize this sensation and let
it know that you see it. If self-care and inner reflection cannot
release an area like this, it is often time to find a good craniosacral
practitioner, or someone from another healing modality, who is
trained to facilitate the release of old trauma.

Once you have a sense of where you are starting out, bring to
mind one of your options. For instance, if you are considering a
job offer, think about the job and what it entails. Imagine yourself
stepping into it. Then ask yourself the following questions:

How do you feel inside?
What changes happen internally?
If you felt some tension initially, does it get tighter or
    does it relax?
Does it feel spacious and light or heavy?

Is there warmth or coolness?
Does a certain color or image show up?
Is it uncomfortable or pleasant?

Pay attention to all the informing your gut, and perhaps the rest of your body, is giving you.

Notice what you think about in response to this information. You may want to write down your sensations and thoughts when you get done to clarify them further.

Take a deep, easy breath, and as you exhale, let go of the option you just considered. Clear your mind.

Now, imagine your other option. Again, take the time to notice all the internal sensations listed above, as well as any thoughts that arise from the deep informing of your inner body wisdom.

This process is one that can be mastered with practice. In important life decisions you may need to return to this inner reflection more than once to get clear about what is optimal for you.

Our life experiences are layered within us, and uncovering what is right can sometimes take days to months to years. Some of my biggest decisions happened in a moment. Others I am still sitting with years after I first asked the question.

Even when long-standing issues do not completely resolve, if you are moving in the best possible direction, it should feel better and better as you go. This is often not an either/or process. There may not be one correct answer.

There are consequences for each decision we make, and being clear about them internally, as well as about the external facts that need to be looked at, is the key to making the optimal decision in any given moment.

Gut Wisdom and Your Health

There are times when you get a clear sense that something is off, like a nagging pain or an ache that won't go away. Your doctor may tell you it is "nothing to worry about," but your gut says not to ignore it. Trust that signal. It can take some detective work on your part, but it is worth it. Paying attention to your body's signals can head a problem off before it becomes a major health issue.

The detective work I am speaking of may also require that you use your integrated gut wisdom. There are so many opportunities for healthcare of all kinds available today. Sometimes bodywork such as CranioSacral Therapy is a good starting place to solve the mystery. Sometimes a body-centered psychotherapy like Somatic Experiencing is what is needed.[4] Acupuncture is another integrative approach that may solve a variety of health issues.

Sometimes the issue is nutritional. It may be that you are missing certain essential nutrients or inadvertently taking in foods that are not good for your body. Finding a good nutritionist or reading the latest research on health and the food you are eating can inform your gut.

This past year I shifted my diet and dropped thirty pounds. I feel like a wet suit several inches thick has been removed from my body. I can move and breathe much more easily. My inner fire is burning brighter. What has made the difference to my health? Eating when I am hungry and stopping when I am full; eating healthy foods that are right for my body type, age, and lifestyle; and listening internally for the signals to guide me. My improved health has also been easy to maintain because the foods I am eating feel right *from the inside out*.

Movement is another major part of health.[5] When we move in ways that nurture us, it can lift depression better than pharmaceuticals, as well as stimulating the flow of nutrients to our cells. Sitting too much has now been found to have detrimental effects almost equal to smoking! In chapter 8, I will speak more about the number of ways movement can help us return to health and stay healthy.

However, the real key to all of these things is that you do

them from a place of sensing that it sits right *in your body*. It may not be easy if you are breaking out of an old pattern, but if you are following your gut knowing, it will ultimately be right for you.

Success Takes Commitment, Courage, and Kindness

This ongoing dialogue with your gut wisdom requires commitment, kindness, and courage, but with practice it will provide you with a deeper sense of inner peace.

Commitment means doing something more than just once or twice when your body wants it every day. That is just a tease that allows your mind to jump in and say, *See, it didn't work*. Make the commitment to continue doing what your body is asking for on a regular schedule. Changing habits isn't easy, so we must stay in the present moment, remain curious, and check in continually with what is needed.[6] Our needs change over time.

On the other hand, commitment can become rigidly rule bound if it is followed beyond what the system is asking for. However, most of us tend to be lax about committing to what is in our best interest, even though it ultimately allows us to give our gifts and share with those we love in a way that we can sustain.

Courage is required because, as any person who has ever been in an unhealthy situation knows, it takes guts and courage to move out of a system or a pattern that is not healthy or life-enhancing. If you are a people-pleasing accommodator, courage is particularly needed. You have probably spent years not listening to your gut (or any other part of your body, for that matter), since survival has meant paying acute attention to what is going on outside of yourself in the lives of others.

An integrated gut helps you take the first steps to moving fully back into the rest of your body as you learn to read the signals about what is right for you, moment to moment.

Finally, kindness to yourself and others is required because none of us do this perfectly. This should be a relief for all the perfectionists out there, afraid that making a mistake or failing at something means disaster for their self-esteem or for their entire life.

Remember, kindness ultimately creates the safety to explore what works best for you in any given moment, and that starts with kindness for yourself. It is astonishing to me the number of people I meet who are kind to others, to animals, to children, and to the environment, but who are really hard on themselves. Kindness has to start at home — in the home of your body.

To access your gut knowing, practice this chapter's exploration. To download the audio, go to www.healingfromthecore.com, click on the Reclaiming Your Body Download link, and enter the password *presence*.

EXPLORATION

The Wisdom of the Gut Exploration

Feel free to do Explorations 1 (pages 55–59) and 2 (pages 59–66) prior to this exploration for a deeper experience. Also remember that Exploration 3 (pages 66 79) is designed to be used whenever you hit a roadblock or some kind of resistance in your Core Embodiment Process — so if, as you are exploring each of the different wisdom areas, you uncover some resistance, that would be an indicator to use Exploration 3 (but certainly not to give up and tell yourself the process simply does not work or docs not work for you).

Inner Awareness

We begin by simply taking a baseline of your inner awareness, without trying to change anything. To do this, allow your feet to rest fully on the floor, eyes closed or semiclosed. As you settle in, following your breath, be curious about the temperature of the air as it enters your nostrils and fills your lungs.

Notice the rise and fall of your chest and back as you breathe normally.

Gut Awareness

Allow yourself to drop your awareness into the area of your gut, from the front of your diaphragm back to your spine and all the way down into the area around your belly button.... Notice what baseline sensations are there when your mind is clear and not contemplating anything in particular. Simply resting your awareness in the present moment.

What informing does your resting gut have for you?

Does it feel like a particular color?

Is it dense or spacious?

Is there a texture to it?

Is there an image or a thought as you breathe and expand your awareness into your entire gut area?

Are you comfortable here?

Is it relaxed or held tight and tense?

We know that a hard, "six pack" flat belly is held up as the ideal in our culture, and yet that does not make for a happy existence...so simply notice where your belly-gut lives on this spectrum from soft and relaxed to hard and tight.

We also know that worries, often old, outdated, but repeated worries can cause your gut to clench.... Notice if your mind is running an inner dialogue of worrying right now and how it is affecting the state of your belly-gut.

Allow yourself to breathe as deeply and easily as you can right down into your belly-gut and feel the rise and fall with each inhale and exhale.

[Pause]

The gut is our most accurate navigator of current-moment danger or rightness in any given situation. This is very different than the way an old worry or fear registers in this area.

So take a moment now and bring to mind some thought process or old worry that you are familiar with in your life...such as being late to an event, or disappointing someone you love, or feeling not good enough in some way....Please do not make it something that overwhelms or devastates you. No tsunamis here!

And as you think about that worry, notice what happens in your gut....Is there a tension registering in your belly-gut right now as you think about that old worry? It may be subtle or big.

Notice the actual physical sensations of it — the charged feeling or the numbness that just showed up, or the density that just increased as you thought about that recurring worry....Pay very close attention to the *sensations* of it and not so much to how your mind responds.

These are sensations that are so frequent that most people take them for granted. They tell themselves, "That's just how my gut feels!" They do not realize there is a cause and effect here when it is coupled with the worrying mind.

Once you have a clear sense of how your gut changed when you started to worry, please let that worry go....Shake it off. Physically shake it off if need be. Get up and move around and come back to your seat if needed.

[Pause]

Then allow yourself to bring to mind a situation that makes you feel safe, happy, and relaxed. See it. Feel it. Breathe it in and notice all the colors and textures of it. Is there a sound that goes with it or a taste or smell?

Notice how your gut reacts to this situation — can you feel it relaxing, letting go, and softening? Give yourself permission to fully experience *this* situation. Notice what happens in the rest of your body as your gut relaxes and softens.

You may notice that when your belly-gut is in this state, it naturally expands down into your legs and feet and on up into your heart and beyond. This state of happiness is the way our belly-gut optimally operates. In fact, feeling truly relaxed and happy is the optimal state for all your cells, not just those in your gut.

Now, please bring to mind a circumstance where something was currently going on around you that was not right. Perhaps the way someone was being treated, or what was being said, or the actions of someone else — but a situation where your gut knew, instinctually, immediately in many cases, that something was wrong....It was off.

How did your gut knowing manifest?

Was it a thought, such as, *Move away from the window* or *Do not take that route?*

Was there an inner uneasiness or some other physical sensation?

Did you hear something?

Did you get an image in your mind's eye that showed you something?

Notice as you register *how* your unique gut knowing manifests...how *these belly-gut sensations are different* from the feelings caused by the old worrisome thought patterns that recycle so frequently.

First, gut knowing happens in the current moment and old fears and worries are...well, old...not happening right now...so allow yourself to really notice the difference.

Also gut knowing is often quiet and uncharged, with a simple sense of knowing it is true, with no fanfare, no drama — simply a sense to take an action or not in the current moment.

And when you are ready, allow yourself to shake off these sensations and return to whatever was helping you feel your safe, relaxed belly-gut, and rest there in your awareness.

Notice how naturally connected a relaxed, open belly-gut is with the rest of your body and with the earth and with the heavens and the air around you.

And enjoy!

7
Your Pelvis
The Gift of Power

*Being aware of your pelvic floor and its intricate connection
to your health is essential to your well-being.*

— KEIRA WETHERUP BROWN

The pelvis, the area in the very bottom of your torso, is a source
of tremendous power, physically as well as emotionally. The
Eastern Vedic traditions speak extensively about the root chakra
and how important it is to the healthy functioning of everything
else in the body. Chinese medicine also honors the pelvis as a major gateway to the body's vital energy flow. However, many people
in Western cultures are ignorant of the importance of this area for
the health of the entire human system.

If the pelvis has been injured, compressed, or compartmentalized, whether due to trauma or cultural/religious issues, it
can have a significant negative effect on long- and short-term
health, as well as diminish the life energy available for creative
endeavors.[1]

Some people are embodied in their pelvic region, but in a
disjointed, compartmentalized manner causing confusion and
disorder.

Pelvic Idioms

She is a pelvic power-
house.
Get your butt in gear.
It was a kick in the
butt.
Feel the sturdiness of
the pelvis.
Gird your loins.
Put your booty in
motion.
It's all about the bass.
Shoot from the hip.
Sit in your power.
The pelvis is the seat
of the soul.
I felt a rumble from
down under.

At the bottom of it all, a return to the embodied wisdom of the pelvis is what naturally fuels creative inspirations, igniting them and you in a good way.

Our sexuality and sensuality as human beings are fueled by this energy as well, and that core energy of who we are is a vital part of living life fully and joyfully.

When we reclaim the energy and wisdom of our pelvis and integrate it with the rest of our body, there is often a marvelous resurgence of life force, bringing a return of desire. Ecstatic experiences can be the outcome of igniting the fire in the pelvis and reuniting it with the legs and feet, gut, heart, voice, and head.

Reclaiming our inner sensations that reside primarily in the pelvis, and linking them to everything else, allows us to feel the deliciousness of being alive. So what gets in the way of reclaiming the pelvis? Often, it is cultural and religious taboos and trauma.

Cultural and Religious Taboos

Body Myth 3 from chapter 2 outlines the issues of growing up in a cultural or religious community where the pelvis and all its energy are completely taboo and seen as seductive or evil — and to be avoided at all costs.

Many religious and spiritual traditions have rigid rules and strict guidelines about how and when the pelvis is acceptable to energetically inhabit and live from, if it is allowed at all! This fact speaks to the power that the pelvis innately radiates and shares when it is healthy and integrated with the rest of the body.

Cultural standards dictate when sex is permissible and with whom. We are given guidelines about how to dress, walk, talk, and give expression to our sensuality and sexuality. Manifestation is either allowed or kept under wraps.

I remember being chastised for self-exploration as a child, not to mention the trouble I got into "playing doctor" with my cousins and siblings. As a young teen I was strictly instructed that sex was not allowed until marriage. If I was to be a "good girl," I must rein in any sensations that might be naturally emanating from that area of my body. Of course, being a typically rebellious teenager, this just piqued my curiosity further.

Based on my experience, I am of the opinion that one reason cultural directives regarding sexuality are so strong and violations so heavily punished is the pelvis is truly *the* engine that fuels our core power and joie de vivre.

A friend of mine, Kelly, grew up in a religious community much like mine, with very strict rules about sexuality. She was an intelligent child, full of enthusiasm for life, who would often sing her heart out in her bedroom with an imaginary microphone. She played the piano endlessly and was involved in the theater when she got to high school.

All of that came to a halt as she matured into a woman and realized that she was sexually attracted to other women. This broke every rule in her parents' rulebook, and she knew the ramifications were damning.

Kelly hid her gender preference, and she definitely kept under wraps her desire for her first love. As she graduated from high school and left for college, she pushed it all down and numbed her pelvis to keep her sanity and be a good daughter.

She became a serious, studious perfectionist about her life and her interests. Upon graduation, Kelly married a gentle, kind man in an effort to convince herself that she was "normal." It did not work, and they divorced several years later.

Kelly's creativity and juice had disappeared along with her

sexual desire. When I met her, she had not belted out a song in decades, much less played the piano. Due to the religious moral code she was raised with, the engine of her body, her pelvis and her sexuality, was forced into hiding.

As she entered her late thirties, Kelly finally openly engaged in relationships with women and told her parents about it. Initially, this devastated them, but she held her ground. When they finally accepted her, it was both liberating and not necessary, since by that point she had already accepted herself.

Then, this past year, an interesting thing happened. Kelly's first love, a sweet woman, came back into her life. In allowing herself to reconnect with her and to love fully and deeply for perhaps the first time in her life, Kelly's inner fire got rekindled. She spontaneously started playing the piano again. She found herself walking around the house singing.

Her pelvis reengaged in ways that she had never allowed before, for fear of reprisal, punishment, and being made an outcast.

Entire civilizations and cultures are run by controlling pelvic power and guiding it in ways that are believed to be right and holy, or simply in order to keep the populace in check.

Truthfully, raw pelvic energy is a force to be reckoned with. If this life force is unintegrated with the rest of the body, it can become quite dangerous. This occurs when the pelvis has been awakened but is compartmentalized and cut off from the rest of the wisdom areas of the body.

Consider Hitler. His power was immense, and he manipulated his impoverished people using well-studied control mechanisms. In a culture beaten down and starving after WWI, he incited people to violence and promised them a return to their own power again.

I highly suspect that Hitler's pelvic energy was distorted and compartmentalized, due to his early childhood shame and trauma. Watch the old movies of the rigid, staccato movements of his military, and you get a peek at the danger in having this powerful engine of the body restricted and only allowed to release in intensely focused ways. Think about the power of an aerosol can and how it will explode if heated, releasing the intense inner pressure in a destructive manner.

Unfortunately, damaged leaders throughout the world have since repeated Hitler's behavior — each time causing fear and chaos and often resulting in destruction and major loss of life.

Trauma and Injury

For almost two decades I have been teaching a course for women entitled "Healing the Pelvic Floor: Reclaiming Your Power, Sexuality, and Pleasure Potential." Trauma is again implicated in the disconnection from our power. Over the years I have seen the debilitating effects of many types of trauma. Trauma from sexual violation or rape is at the top of the list.

In her landmark book *Vagina*, Naomi Wolf explores the ramifications to a woman's spirit and general life force when the pelvis is severely damaged, such as what occurs in the repeated rape and violation of women in wartime.[2]

Having a baby can be traumatic due to the business of birthing in our medical system. Surgery for the bladder, colon, and reproductive organs can cause pain or numbness, significantly diminishing the ability to feel pleasure at all.

For a woman, verbal or emotional abuse by her family, religion, or culture can cause such disempowerment that she may believe she has no right to drop into her own pelvis and harness her innate power.

Men who suffer trauma from sexual abuse or violence to their pelvic region may experience diminished power and capability in the world as well. Violence to a man's pelvic area or shaming for his genital size can create withdrawal from this area of the body, leaving him depleted and numb. For young men in gangs, trauma is endemic, due to their violent, often sexual initiations and lifestyle.

Ultimately, any unresolved trauma in the pelvis will cause a diminishment of energy and thus of power for anyone.

Healing Partners — The Pelvis and the Heart

The antidote to pelvic trauma, regardless of the cause, is not to control or suppress this area, but to heal it. Only then can this natural power source be harnessed and connected to the rest of the system, which it is meant to fuel.

When the gut's insight, which signals us when something is either right or wrong, is connected to the pelvis's power and the heart's wisdom, there is a deep integrity that is innate to all of us as human beings. Add the grounding of feeling your legs and feet, and the clarity of your bones' intelligence, and only then does your mind have all the information it needs to make wise, clear decisions.

In particular, the heart's naturally emerging inspiration needs the energy of the pelvis to be able to bring it to fruition — to completion. Of course, the pelvis needs the heart as a guiding force to channel its energy in ways that are good for the whole system and for others.

A perfect example of someone badly in need of this partnership is Jeannine, a college friend. Jeannine is a wonderful, creative person who is full of ideas and talent. She is constantly expanding into her *next* artistic adventure. The problem is she never follows through in ways that allow her to bring her ideas to completion. It is as though her heart is full and brimming over with inspiration, which quickly dissipates. Her home is filled with collections of uncompleted projects. She appears to have no steady energy source to help her ground and manifest her artistic dreams.

I have seen this pattern repeatedly in others when the power of the pelvis is missing in action.

Another pattern that I have seen is when the pelvis has sustained trauma and is depleted or diminished in its capacities, but the person pushes themselves using their will. This may be due to a perceived or real need to keep going, even though the pelvis, the engine of the body, is not functioning well. This situation creates a double whammy because it depletes other systems in the body in the drive to make things happen, even though the best action is to rest, heal, and bring the whole system into balance.

Not Pausing to Heal

Sarah is a vibrant, talented woman who fell and broke her coccyx in a skiing accident. She could not sit down without extreme pain for a month, and even when the pain dissipated, the dull ache would show up whenever she sat for too long in one position.

Despite this, Sarah kept going in her life. Sarah told me, "I just numbed out below the waist in order to keep up with my schedule — my kids, my job, and my relationship with my husband."

Sarah's sexual energy became vastly diminished, and her overall energy was much lower. She felt irritable in a way that had never been true before. She had always prided herself on being easygoing and flexible. Now when her kids or her husband asked her for something, since her energy reservoir was so low, she felt like saying, "If you ask me for one more thing…"

A friend suggested Sarah see me, and when she finally arrived on my treatment table, a year had passed since the accident and her overall health was becoming affected. Her natural resilience was gone. She said, "My immune system is on vacation, and I badly need one, too."

I asked her how much time she had taken off after the accident, and I was shocked when she said she had not stopped at all. She said her life was too full to rest. People depended on her. She felt she could not stop. I know this is a common theme in the lives of many parents and caregivers and overly burdened professionals of all kinds. It certainly seems valid given the pace of our lives. Yet the body suffers the consequences when this occurs — especially with injuries to this "engine" area of the body.

When I took her sacrum in my hand, it felt dense and compressed. It was not moving in the normal craniosacral rhythm. I asked her to allow her awareness to drop into this area, and it was almost impossible for her to do so. She felt thin threads of sensation but could not sustain it. Her story of how hard and painful the last year had been came pouring out.

When I gently asked her if there was a reason she hadn't stopped to let the coccyx heal, she began to cry. She had lived her life meeting the demands of and pleasing others. She truthfully had no idea how to switch gears. The idea of curtailing some of her responsibilities in order to heal seemed impossible.

As I reminded her that there was no time like the present moment to change that habit, I felt a sense of warmth seeping into her lower back and sacrum. The tight holding she had been doing for the last year to keep it all together was letting go. Minutes passed, and we both sensed a growing warmth and relaxation there.

Once this occurred, I could release her sacrum and coccyx from the compressed, twisted position it was caught in. Immediately, heat from her pelvis flooded up her spine and throughout her torso. Her legs relaxed as well. Her chest and face turned a rosy pink color. She started to giggle, and before long we were laughing full-out. The laughter freed up the rest of her system.

This was the case of a woman who desperately wanted to heal, but she just didn't understand what to do to get there. Sarah's life continues to change as she recognizes the energy she lost and then regained from the release of her pelvis in this session. Because the injury was so serious, she is still working to maintain the changes we achieved, and she regularly practices the exploration below, "The Wisdom of the Pelvis-Heart Connection." Sarah is learning to listen to her body signals in order to maintain a full energy reservoir.

To regain your pelvic energy and harness it in partnership with your heart and deepest inspirations, practice this chapter's exploration. To download the audio, go to www.healing-fromthecore.com, click on the Reclaiming Your Body Download link, and enter the password *presence*.

EXPLORATION

The Wisdom of the Pelvis-Heart Connection Exploration

Feel free to do Explorations 1 (pages 55–59) and 2 (pages 59–66) prior to this exploration for a deeper experience. Also remember that Exploration 3 (pages 66–79) is designed to be used whenever you hit a roadblock or some kind of resistance in your Core Embodiment Process — so if, as you are exploring each of the different wisdom areas, you uncover some resistance, that would be an indicator to use Exploration 3 (but certainly not to give up and tell yourself the process simply does not work or does not work for you).

Inner Awareness

We begin by simply taking a baseline of your inner awareness, without trying to change anything. To do this, allow your feet to rest fully on the floor, eyes closed or semiclosed. As you settle in, following your breath, be curious about the temperature of the air as it enters your nostrils and fills your lungs.

Notice the sensations of your spine being supported by your chair, and the rise and fall of your belly with each inhale and exhale.

Pelvis Awareness

Allow your awareness to drop down into your pelvis...your reproductive system and pelvic floor...your sacrum and coccyx, as you breathe, inhaling and exhaling...dropping deeper and deeper, into the engine of your body.

What are the sensations that arise here?

Does it feel warm or cool?

Is there a color, a texture?

Does it feel open and connected to your gut and heart?

The questions answered by this wisdom area are, "Do I have access to my power? Am I standing in my power? Do I *have* the power to support what the rest of me needs and wants?"

Just notice the response from your pelvis to these questions....

Is this natural well of energy open and functioning?

This area will also inform you if the strength is or is not there at this time.

In any case, take a moment now and drop your awareness from your pelvis down through your legs and feet into the earth, making that safe, unconditional connection, as deeply into the earth as you feel comfortable with right now.

[Pause]

As you breathe, allow your feet and legs to fill with nurturing sensations and energy....As this river of nourishment reaches your pelvis, allow the bones of your pelvis to soak up these sensations like a dry sponge soaking in clear water...filling and energizing, relaxing and opening to what would nurture you most in this moment.

Is it warm or cool?

Does it have a particular color or texture?

As your bones fill, allow this river of safe nourishment to soak into your organs and organ systems here in this area...energizing your cells as it feeds them...awakening your awareness as they fill.

Notice how your pelvis feels now as it fills and connects with your belly-gut and then on into your heart....The pelvis, gut, and heart are meant to be partnered when decision making is pending or life is challenging.

Your heart and gut offer your pelvis moment-by-moment guidance and shepherd this powerful engine so it does not go astray from what would be best or optimal for the entire system.

Notice how your pelvis feels, supported by your legs and feet ...and the earth.

[Pause]

And how your gut and heart feel supported by your pelvis and the ground.

Good....Allow your awareness to return to just your pelvis and notice what informing it may have for you right now, as it is connected, supported, and teamed up with the other areas of the body.

Are there any images, colors, textures, or knowing of some other kind emanating from this hopefully powerful engine of who you are?

If you are an overly optimistic dreamer, it may signal you to regroup or slow down what you are doing. This accurate energy "reality check" is one of the gifts that the pelvis has for you.

If you are headed in a direction that is right for you, your pelvis may give you a full "go ahead" signal if the energy is there, which can ignite your dreams and inspirations and help you take the next step to manifesting them.

And breathing deeply into your pelvis, thank it for the experience you have just had, and allow your awareness to expand back out into the world around you.

And enjoy!

8

Your Legs and Feet
The Gift of Movement

*If you don't have answers to your problems after a four-hour run,
you ain't getting them.*

— CHRISTOPHER McDOUGALL

One of the marvels of the human body is what I call the metabolizing effect of our legs and feet when they are activated. Beyond that function, they have an inner intelligence as well, which you will see below.

Legs and Feet Help Us Metabolize

This wisdom area of the body is one that helps us take what we experience as confusing, disorienting, or simply puzzling and metabolize it — digest it. I don't mean this in the literal sense of breaking down our food into substances that can nourish us, but in the metaphoric sense of finding clarity about our lives, our challenges, our biggest questions.

When I was younger, I was a runner. Now I walk and walk and walk. Whenever I have an issue or a problem, I walk it out —

Legs and Feet Idioms

He didn't have a leg
to stand on.

She is standing tall.

I was cut off at the
knees.

We are stepping out
tonight.

It's like walking a mile
in his shoes.

He thinks she's the
bee's knees.

He was brought to his
knees.

She was on her last
legs.

Getting sea legs takes
time.

He has to cool his
heels.

Don't dig in your
heels.

He was keeping her
on her toes.

He stepped on their
toes in that
situation.

She was fleet of foot.

She dragged her feet
on that issue.

He found his footing
after all.

Getting your feet wet
is important.

or "metabolize" it. I head out on the path without thinking about what I am trying to figure out, and most days by the end of the walk the answer appears.

My friend Bobbi, a talented pediatric therapist, informs me that the Brain Gym curriculum teaches how moving our limbs in a cross-body motion stimulates and integrates the hemispheres of the brain.[1]

Any physical activity, like taking a walk or a run, facilitates integration between the body and the brain — as long as our limbs move in a synchronized manner. Thus, by doing this kind of exercise, tissues in areas that are stuck or caught can start moving again.

Also, think about what happens to people when they are frozen with trauma. Often people who have sustained traumatic injuries that were overwhelming go into a contracted or dissociated, frozen place, and a felt sense of one's legs and feet are one of the first things to disappear. When this occurs, the healing process is stymied.

Stimulating small movements can end stasis at a cellular level. Full-body movements help to heal overall frozen shock states, and both are the antidote needed for healing trauma at a core level. And nothing is more nonthreatening than taking a walk!

One review of research done by Harvard showed that daily aerobic exercise lifts mild to moderate depressive symptoms by 60 to 70 percent, which was equal to the effectiveness of antidepressant medications (like the SSRI Zoloft).[2] Further, exercisers maintained their gains longer than those on antidepressants as long as they continued to move their legs and feet regularly in an aerobic manner.

One study found that walking fast for about thirty-five minutes a day for five times a week, or sixty minutes a day for three times per week, had a significant influence on moderate depression. This bestows all the health benefits of exercise in terms of the mood-lifting effects of endorphins, enhanced immune function, and reduction of pain perception.

Also, think about how muddled and overwhelming it can feel to deal with stressful situations that have a lot of options. After traumatic events, and even with normal stressors, we know that our perceptual lens is narrowed and our ability to come up with creative solutions is vastly reduced.

She got her foot in the door.
He had a foot in both camps.
He has feet of clay.
I've got itchy feet to leave.
That old man has one foot in the grave.
He was back on his feet.
I was following in her footsteps.
We are footloose and fancy-free.
Get a foothold.
Don't get off on the wrong foot.
He went down on bended knee.
This news story has legs.
He landed on his feet after that disaster.
She got cold feet about the wedding.

When we get moving and activate our legs and feet to sort it all out, the potential for excellent healing solutions is immense — if we can remember to use them!

Josh, a good friend, faced a difficult decision as to whether or not to proceed with a complicated prostate surgery. He had researched his options thoroughly, but no definitive answer emerged. His issues were in a "gray zone" with no clear statistics to support one direction or the other.

Pressure mounted as the deadline approached for his decision. The amount of data was overwhelming, and he was at an impasse despite his superior analytical skills.

As Josh described it: "At the eleventh hour, I instinctively threw on my coat and headed out the door. I walked and walked, thinking about everything and nothing. All the statistical data was forgotten as I put one foot in front of the other. When I rounded the corner to return home, I realized that something had shifted inside me, and I was no longer confused."

Josh had "metabolized" all the data, and as he completed his walk, he had a clear solution. He followed through with his decision, and the surgery was completely successful.

I recently ran across another clear example of this.

World-renowned writer and speaker Gregg Braden tells the story of a particularly difficult decision he made in November 1997 about whether to take a tour of forty people to Egypt right after a terrorist attack.[3] Known as "the Luxor Massacre," the attack killed fifty-eight tourists and four Egyptians. Braden credits his deep heart's knowing with helping him make the decision to go ahead with the tour.

However, his story also speaks to the wisdom of the legs and feet:

> Immediately I began receiving phone calls regarding the planned tour. Family and friends begged me not to go. The people signed up for the trip begged me not to cancel. The Egyptian authorities were concerned about the possibility of another attack. And the tour company was waiting for me to make a decision and do so quickly....I felt pulled from all sides. Everyone I spoke with had an opinion, and they all made perfect sense....Clearly, this

was one of those times when the decision was not black-and-white; there was no right or wrong and no way of knowing what would happen over the course of the following days and weeks. There was only me, my instincts, my intuition, and my promise to honor my group and myself with the best choice possible.

Overwhelmed by the chaos of information and opinions, I turned off the telephone and shut off the input from other people. From my home in the high desert of northern New Mexico, *I went for a long walk down a dirt road that I have visited many times in the past when I had to make a tough decision* [italics added].

Braden returned from that walk with the decision to proceed as planned. The trip was an incredible success in multiple ways.

His heart's intelligence clearly made a good decision for all in this case, *with the support and wisdom of his legs and feet*, which were engaged during that walk.

The wisdom that comes from activating our legs and feet is often ignored. Yet they are ready and waiting to be a powerful support if we can only remember to utilize it in such moments, as Gregg Braden did without realizing it or even thinking about it!

Our Legs and Feet Are Smart

Let's take this a level deeper, beyond what occurs when we activate our legs and feet by moving them. There is innate intelligence or knowing that resides in this area of the body.

When we are not paying attention to or are unable to feel the sensations in our feet and legs, we cannot benefit from the deep informing that emerges from them.

Our legs and feet are not merely the "workhorses" of our bodies to be whipped into shape. They are powerful allies helping us discern *how* to move forward with our lives. Whether the message is "Get moving!" or "Slow down!" their wisdom is always there if we can learn to tune in and receive the wisdom we seek.

One client, Joan, is a great example of this. Joan found her way to me after a critical illness forced changes in her professional life. By the time we met, she had recovered from her illness, left her job, and moved on with her life. She was developing skills in other arenas more gratifying for her.

However, the effects of that challenging time period had shaken her deeply and were lingering in her body, robbing her of peace of mind and clarity. Joan's session began with her explaining how she needed help embracing and moving forward with her healing gifts.

"I love using my gifts in the work I am doing," she said. "My clients love it, too. I feel energized. So why am I still feeling tentative about building my practice?"

As she dropped her awareness deep into her body, Joan was drawn all the way down into her feet. She realized she felt as though she had one foot on the accelerator and the other foot on the brake. No wonder she had difficulty moving forward in terms of manifesting her gifts more fully.

Whenever she would step into a new endeavor, no matter how right it felt (accelerating her dreams), she found herself slipping into self-doubt and slamming on the brakes. She was in a cycle of self-sabotage.

Joan shared: "I feel cautious in the last few years, since that time of my burning out and getting so ill. That time period was such a difficult ride for me. My boundaries were nearly nonexistent. I lived on high alert, overfunctioning all the time, and yet I could not keep up with the needs of my constituents. I can still remember the deep clenching in my gut that preceded the illness that almost killed me."

When I suggested that she check in with the sensations in her legs and feet, Joan was astounded. "Oh my God, they were telling me to slow down the whole time, but I was oblivious. I was focused on my need to please everyone else."

I asked if she still had a tendency to do too much. Joan chuckled and told me that her inner "perfectionist" was *sure* she has not done enough. However, her friends and colleagues told her she ran circles around them.

Joan went on: "In my head, I know that I do way more than the average person, but somehow the message has not gotten through to that old part of me that is sure that *I am not quite enough.*"

"What is the effect on your legs and feet of feeling like you are not doing enough?" I asked her quietly.

"I feel pressure building up again as though my heels are digging in." Then she laughed. "My feet and legs are saying, *Hell, no! We won't go!* I have literally dug in my heels. My legs and feet are still afraid I will throw myself into my work, lose my boundaries, and burn out all over again."

After a good laugh, we returned to the sensations in her legs and feet. She was noticing, she said, that "my feet and legs are firmly held as if in concrete, absolutely determined not to move. Yet the creative part of me is stretching in a dozen different directions and feeling exhausted. This gives a whole new meaning to the phrase *stretched too thin!*"

I asked her, "What would it feel like if you could give yourself a message like 'I do plenty right now.' Or, 'What I do is enough.'"

Her response was immediate. "When I tell myself that, the deep pressure eases up!"

I asked: "What do your feet and legs need in order to take the brakes off so they can work with the rest of you?"

An image emerged in Joan's mind. She saw herself sitting quietly every day and checking in with her legs and feet about her plans for the day. She already regularly practiced the Core

Embodiment Process, but somehow the wisdom of her legs and feet kept getting left out.

"I feel my feet, but I have not been communicating with them regularly. I had no idea that they had information like this for me," Joan said.

As it turned out, her feet and legs were quite a comical conversation partner. Joan chuckled and said, "They are saying to me, *That's right, sister, and notice all we do for you every day! You, Ms. High and Mighty, listening to your head and your heart — what are we, chopped liver?*"

We were both roaring with laughter at this last communication. Joan reassured her legs and feet that she had them firmly in her sights and would ask them, "What is ours to do today, legs and feet?" She would add them to her inner team for all future discussions and decisions.

As the session came to a close, Joan received a new mantra, "Feet First." She could feel her heart relax as her legs and feet knew they were heard and seen, and more energy flowed through them into the rest of her body. I applauded her feet for holding their ground until Joan could figure out the message they were sending.

Joan thanked her legs and feet. She took a moment to check in with the rest of her system. Her heart felt deeply inspired by her work. Today, Joan has learned how to have balance and healthy boundaries. She knows how to take care of herself first, *then* share her gifts from a full, centered place.

Joan realized that including her feet and legs in her decision making leads to a happy heart and helps her make wise choices about all the things in her life. They help her focus, not just on pleasing others, but on truly satisfying herself.

Creativity and Beyond

Beyond metabolizing and problem solving, our legs and feet are a wisdom area that also stimulates brainstorming capacity. For instance, a 2014 study found that people who walked for eight minutes produced ideas that were rated as 61 percent more creative than those of people who simply sat during that time.[4]

Whether it is the right- and left-brain integration, or some other mechanism, that is responsible for this kind of increase in creativity, it is worth remembering when you are brainstorming or wanting to open to new horizons creatively. This wisdom is called for when there are many sides to an issue, and layers of complexity to deal with, in any given idea, quest, or inspiration — perplexing problems to be solved, barriers to be met and dissolved. When this occurs, as is often the case in our lives, the wisdom of the legs and feet are needed.

This wisdom area is often overlooked because we are such a left-brain, heady culture. However, it is such a valuable asset to who we are as integrated, creative human beings. In fact, the best way to activate the wisdom of the legs and feet is to get them moving, as in take a walk, a run, a swim, or any other form of rhythmic, synchronized movement.

However, if or when that is not possible, then the following exploration will activate the wisdom of your legs and feet. This chapter's exploration will help you embody more deeply this area of your body. To download the audio, go to www.healingfromthecore.com, click on the Reclaiming Your Body Download link, and enter the password *presence*.

EXPLORATION

The Wisdom of the Legs and Feet Exploration

Feel free to do Explorations 1 (pages 55–59) and 2 (pages 59–66) prior to this exploration for a deeper experience. Also remember that Exploration 3 (pages 66–79) is designed to be used whenever you hit a roadblock or some kind of resistance in your Core Embodiment Process — so if, as you are exploring each of the different wisdom areas, you uncover some resistance, that would be an indicator to use Exploration 3 (but certainly not to give up and tell yourself the process simply does not work or does not work for you).

Inner Awareness

We begin by simply taking a baseline of your inner awareness, without trying to change anything. To do this, allow your feet to rest fully on the floor, eyes closed or semiclosed. As you settle in, following your breath, be curious about the temperature of the air as it enters your nostrils and fills your lungs.

Legs and Feet Awareness

Bring to mind a question or issue in your life to which you do not currently have an answer. Or perhaps you have many possibilities. Recognize them. Thank them for showing up, and then ask them to rest back in your consciousness for a bit.

Then imagine yourself taking a walk with this issue, dropping down into your legs and on down into your feet, breathing and stimulating the desire to move forward on this deep inspiration. The wisdom of our legs and feet is designed to help us with integrating the whole process.

In your mind's eye, take this walk somewhere that's beautiful for you so that your attention is on the scenery, and you can let everything "digest" without thinking about it.

Imagine yourself walking at a comfortable pace, swinging your arms, your heart pumping. As this occurs, effortlessly it metabolizes or digests the issue you are mulling over. This cross-body movement integrates the right and left hemispheres of your brain as well as moving this knowing throughout the rest of your system.

When you're ready, let your walk come to an end and notice what new information or answers appear in your consciousness.

And enjoy!

9 Your Bones
The Gifts of Clarity and Steadiness

That inner voice has both gentleness and clarity.
So to get to authenticity, you really keep going down to the bone,
to the honesty, and the inevitability of something.

— MEREDITH MONK

Our bones offer us a particular kind of wisdom that is vital in today's chaotic, sometimes overwhelming world. It is the gift of being able to feel steady when emotions are overwhelming as well as the gift of being able to see things clearly when issues feel muddy and confusing.

"I knew it deep in my bones" is a favorite idiom that connotes a knowing that comes from a clear, strong place that will not waver.

The ramifications of being in our bones, particularly in times of turmoil, are that we can become an oasis of calm, a beacon of clear light, when the world feels murky.

Yet we are generally not taught this as children. We are for the most part taught how to pay attention to the external world, constantly seeking approval and connection. In order to do this, we frequently learn how to suppress emotion, rather than process it in a healthy way. Or we live feeling overwhelmed by our emotions and inner signals, not knowing how to be with and process it all.

Think back to the story I tell in chapter 1: how when I hurt my finger, my father needed me to stop crying. I sensed that and suppressed my fears and tears, which I was in the process of releasing. I know now that my emotional state was probably causing my father some inner anxiety. Being the good daughter that I was, I discounted my pain and stopped crying prematurely.

What if my father had been able to be a steady presence that calmed me and allowed my fear and pain to come to a natural healing close?

Wouldn't you prefer to be *that* presence for those around you?

The Steady, Calm Presence of Our Bones

What I have seen repeatedly is that when someone holds that steady, calm presence, it helps everyone else in the vicinity come to that place more quickly within themselves. So how does this work?

Our bones are the sturdiest, densest part of our anatomy, our connective tissue, forming the scaffolding — the structure — that supports everything else.

When we can embody in our bones — when we can take our awareness into these innermost chambers of who we are — a quality of steadiness naturally emanates from them. Whatever emotions we are caught up in are then held gently for a natural resolution.

In chapter 2, I tell the story of Jennifer, who dissolved into tears during the opening of a class as she shared her history. In that moment, I utilized the gift of helping her feel the steadiness of her bones to help her gain her inner equilibrium and hold that huge ball of pain she had arrived with. As she followed my simple directions, she settled easily in her bones and could hold and process with more grace and ease.

In traditional Chinese acupuncture, the bones are considered a water element, among the five elements of fire, air, water, earth, and wood. The season of the water element is winter, when we are naturally meant to go inward, to rest in quiet, refilling and rejuvenating from the deep well of our bone marrow. This is why bone broth soup is so often recommended for recovery and healing from severe illness and bone breaks. When we have good bone energy, Chinese medicine teaches us that we have an inner reservoir, which provides resilience and a capacity to roll with what life offers us, rather than being overwhelmed by it.

Furthermore, when you drop into your bones and rest there, it offers clarity, as we now inhabit our deepest recesses, rather than being buffeted around and confused by external demands. One of the things I see is that it helps us know what we need and what we want in our lives with more precision and surety.

Sometimes this clarity brings information forward that we would rather not see. Recently, when I did this chapter's bone wisdom exploration with a client, he shared that what came into crystal-clear focus was the extent of his Lyme disease. This was not a pleasant awareness or sensation, but it helped him choose

Bones Idioms

I'm bone-tired.
He doesn't have a serious bone in his body.
I knew it deep in my bones.
She's good to the bone.
I have a bone to pick.
She was the backbone of the organization.
Every bone in my body wanted that.
I worked my fingers to the bone.
That issue is the main bone of contention.
What's in your bone pile?
That remark cut me to the bone.
That's close to the bone.

the next therapeutic routes to try. And he was not feeling over-whelmed by this knowledge — just aware of the extent of his issue.

Clarity and steadiness are two of the main gifts of our bones.

Losing Touch with Our Bones

Many people are overaccommodating. They take care of everyone else's needs before their own. In doing so, they often lose track of how they feel inside. The natural consequence of living a life that is constantly outwardly focused is that we can miss learning the skills for how to know what we need internally. Many women are raised to take care of others, and ignore themselves, and many men are also raised this way. Though men provide for others in a different way, they often do so at the expense of their own inner-most health and well-being.

Unresolved trauma is another reason people frequently miss the gift that our bones give us. When someone has suffered trauma, and it remains lodged in the body or mind unprocessed, the brain is constantly on alert for anything that looks, smells, tastes, or sounds like the original trauma. This brilliant survival mechanism keeps us from making the same mistake twice. The problem is that we can spend our life, often unconsciously, on red alert, always focused *externally* while searching the horizon for danger.

This form of hypervigilance is not only depleting, as it takes a lot of energy to keep this up, but it also leaves very little time or attention for knowing ourselves *internally*. Our bones are our in-nermost recesses, and they are the first casualty of our awareness when it is split between the external and the internal. Survival always comes first. Hypervigilance says: Let me pay attention to my own needs later, when I can finally relax and let down. The problem is that this softening into life rarely comes without some form of healing to resolve the trauma memories. When that occurs, then it's easier to learn how to live from deep within.

Too Much Stability

What about people who seem so overly grounded they are like the Rock of Gibraltar? Aren't they the epitome of bone-deep wisdom presence? Not really.

When someone has been taught to be the stabilizing force in a given system — such as a family or an organization — they may do so in a manner that locks them inside that role, so that they are unable to see what is actually happening outside of themselves in terms of their own health and well-being.

This can happen due to illness in a family or lack of resources. By becoming overly stabilized, the person loses the information that comes with fluidity and being open to the changes that are healthy for us.

George is a prime example of this. When he first came to me, his wife had recently died after a decade-long battle with cancer. He had been the stabilizing force the whole time, for her and their two children. He was starting to feel the effects on his own health, while not really understanding the underlying dynamic of his depletion.

George came to me because one of his friends recommended that he do so, but according to George himself, he was fine. He had done an excellent job of being the Rock of Gibraltar in his family and extended circles. He was well loved by everyone he knew. He just had a hard time letting in their care and concern.

This is one of the characteristics of those who overstabilize. The metaphoric "receiving buttons" are turned off. Yet life is meant to be a balance of both receiving and giving nurturing, nourishing connection. When more goes out than comes in, people are there for everyone else but not for themselves.

In our sessions together, I explained this concept to George as I gently held his tight, tense spine with open, flat hands, which acted like energy baskets he could rest back into when he was ready.

Speaking quietly to his spine, I recognized how it had "held it all together" for his family all those years. I asked his muscles and bones, cradled in my hands, how it felt having done such an admirable job for such a long time. The first small wave of relaxation arrived after those words sank in.

Then, for the first time, his body registered the exhaustion he was feeling. I asked if it wanted to let go some more. George's immediate response was, "I can't. Who will hold it all together if I let go and relax?"

Gently, I reminded George that the worst was over. He had made it to the finish line with his late wife. Now, in the aftermath of her death, his extended family and community were there for both him and his teenage children.

In fact, his body had not registered that — it was still frozen in that overstabilizing position, even though it was no longer appropriate or needed.

As George realized what was happening in the present moment, his tissues began to relax even more. It was as though, with the aid of my nurturing touch, he was updating his internal operating system.

Tears of relief trickled from his eyes as he let go, layer by layer, into my hands. His entire backbone and musculature felt like it was melting — in a good way. Although he was technically in his bones the whole time, in fact, he was frozen there, unable to move to do anything but care for others.

This is a noble and compassionate role to choose. However, when we are frozen there, it can be very detrimental to our health and well-being.

As we finished up his session, his entire body felt much more relaxed. He could sense what was going on inside in a much deeper way. The smile on his face said it all.

I knew that with his new internal awareness, his navigational system could now register more clearly what direction he needed to move in for the health and well-being of himself and his family. We spoke about that in our final minutes together, and he left feeling like he had gotten the proverbial "new lease on life."

Hiding Out in Your Bones

Another way in which someone can be present in their bones, but not in a healthy manner, is when they have contracted deep inside as a stress or trauma response. Just like the stress response of dissociating or leaving one's body, this contracted state causes the person to lose touch with or have less sensation within. I see it as a "hunkering down inside" in order to survive a threat of some kind.

It is like someone retreating behind the walls of a castle and closing the gate — no new information gets in — and much of what comes out is not appropriate to the present time. This person is often living out of memories and making decisions from outdated patterns and ideas. This is not a healthy boundary, although it may have originally been an attempt at having a boundary in an overwhelming situation, which made sense at the time.

The key in healing this kind of pattern is first to acknowledge the contracted state as a successful strategy for survival in a bad situation. If you are talking to and holding space for someone in this state, his or her very presence is evidence of the success of the strategy. They survived!

Nurturing touch can be introduced to the healing process when appropriate. Touch is a primary locator for people, one of the most powerful, effective ways to help someone come into the present moment of sensation.

Touch and Awareness Are Powerful Antidotes

In many, many sessions I have gently held someone's shoulders, spine, or sacrum, their knees or feet. I do this until, using my noninvasive touch as a locator, the person's awareness returns to these areas — anywhere in the body that makes a connection to the person's bones will work. When that bone-deep knowing happens, the person often spontaneously comes out with what they need or want, even though moments earlier they had no clue. This process can take a few minutes, or it may need to be repeated over days. The key is sensing deep within the bones and resting there until that quiet clarity arrives.

For people with trauma, touch — this powerful but gentle form of connection — can be the first step in healing the unresolved issues within, so that they can return home to themselves.

However, the kind of touch used and how it proceeds must be done carefully. Many people who have survived deep trauma mistakenly think that they need deep or invasive touch to reach these contracted places inside themselves. These clients fill massage therapists' offices wanting deep-tissue work that borders on being retraumatizing at times.

More times than I can count, my clients with this contracted survival pattern have come into my office telling me about a new therapy that someone recommended. It involved touch, sounds, or movement (or some combination) that was powerful and invasive, "but in a good way," they say.

When I ask them to describe the process, they admit that it was a *bit* overwhelming, and it caused pain, but they explain, "The therapist told me that was good for me — I am sure it was part of the releasing process of what has been so bound down." However, when I put my hands on the person, the tissue has recoiled into a tighter pattern than before. Or progress we had made in previous sessions has disappeared.

Upon further inquiry, people admit that while they originally bought the idea that this therapy could help them break through and heal quicker — perhaps once and for all — it actually left them limping, contracted, or disoriented for some time afterward. In other words, the "therapeutic work" was retraumatizing.

What works best, in my experience, is to hold a gentle nurturing touch that feels noninvasive to the receiver. Then you allow the person being touched to bring their awareness out of their contracted frozen place to meet you. This may take time, and it requires a sense of safety and therapeutic presence from the therapist.

The noninvasive release techniques of CranioSacral Therapy really shine here, as they free up the physical restrictions that can result from trauma of all kinds. This allows the body-mind-spirit to have more internal connection and awareness as the nervous system operates more optimally.

To embody more deeply in your own bones, follow the steps in this chapter's exploration. To download the audio, go to www .healingfromthecore.com, click on the Reclaiming Your Body Download link, and enter the password *presence*.

EXPLORATION

The Wisdom of the Bones Exploration

Feel free to do Explorations 1 (pages 55–59) and 2 (pages 59–66) prior to this exploration for a deeper experience. Also remember that Exploration 3 (pages 66–79) is designed to be used whenever you hit a roadblock or some kind of resistance in your Core Embodiment Process — so if, as you are exploring each of the different wisdom areas, you uncover some resistance, that would be an indicator to use Exploration 3 (but certainly not to give up and tell yourself the process simply does not work or does not work for you).

Inner Awareness

We begin by simply taking a baseline of your inner awareness, without trying to change anything. To do this, allow your feet to rest fully on the floor, eyes closed or semiclosed. As you settle in, following your breath, be curious about the temperature of the air as it enters your nostrils and fills your lungs.

Notice the rise and fall of your chest and back as you breathe normally.

Bones Awareness

Next, allow your awareness to drop into your bones, deep into your innermost recesses — those sturdy, steady parts of who you are. Your bones are your densest, strongest connective tissue, and most of them exist deep in the core of your body. They form the structure upon which everything else rests.

And yet even as they are sturdy and strong, they also have air spaces like sponges do — or we would all weigh a whole lot more! So allow yourself to sense or see or feel these wonderful air spaces that are a part of your bones.

And as you imagine them, allow yourself to drop more deeply inside by riding your inhalation, your in-breath, right into those air spaces, and as you exhale allowing your awareness to rest deep inside.

On the next inhale, going deeper; on the next exhale, resting deep in the inner sanctum of your bones. You can enter all of them as you breathe...or choose one area that suits you best. It might be your spine, or the bones of your pelvis, or your legs and feet. Wherever it feels easy to sink into in this moment, and rest there with your attention deep inside of you.

Take a pause now to sit in silence with your awareness deep inside, noticing the clarity that comes as the mud of your life's activities settles and you sit deeper in the calmness your bones naturally provide.

[Pause]

Take as long as you need to feel the steadying, clear sense that this wisdom area provides. Notice the deep informing coming from your bones.

[Pause]

And when you are ready, allow your awareness to expand out into all the rest of you, infusing your cells with the calm, steady clarity of your bones' wisdom.

And enjoy!

10

Your Brain
The Gifts of
an Integrated System

Follow your heart but take your brain with you.

— ALFRED ADLER

For centuries the Western educated world has subscribed to a "top down" theory where the brain is concerned. Descartes's famous phrase "I think, therefore I am" says it all. According to this conceptual framework, what goes on between the ears is the master, and everything below the neck is the servant.

In the last two decades, this long-held theory has been challenged from many directions. The 1990s brought a new focus in neuroscience research. Innovative methods of brain scans and monitoring brought to light the complexity of our entire human system.

New information is coming forward indicating that much of what goes on in our brains originates from signals, beyond normal physiological functioning, sent by the heart, the gut, the pelvis, and probably other areas yet to be discovered by scientific research. Intelligence, previously believed to originate only in the brain, is now understood to also arise from what I call the wisdom areas of the body.

The brain is a very important member of the team that makes up our whole human system. However, it is not the all-powerful boss it was previously thought to be.

Having said that, several areas of the brain are known to be important for processing signals and information coming in from the different areas of the body.

The prefrontal cortex is one such area — it's located directly behind your forehead, behind and above your eyes.[1] Anatomically, this area includes the anterior cingulate cortex, the orbitofrontal cortex, the medial prefrontal (dorsal and ventral sides) cortex, and the ventrolateral prefrontal cortex.

When this area of the brain is healthy, connected, and operating optimally, the prefrontal cortex registers and processes a wide number of things, from morality to fear modulation to emotional balance and insight. It organizes and then strategizes using the powerful information coming in moment to moment from our body. Signals coming in from all our senses as well as the wisdom areas of the body give the brain the information to make decisions and instigate actions.

The prefrontal cortex *is associated with* or *mediates* the processes I describe below. What we know is that, if there is damage to these areas due to physical or emotional trauma, these functions will be impaired. We also know that many forms of meditation and the work I present in this book can and does strengthen the prefrontal function.

Let's take a closer look at what the latest research shows.[2]

Body Regulation

When the parasympathetic arm of the nervous system (the rest-and-digest function) and the sympathetic arm (the accelerator that helps us respond to stressors) are balanced appropriately, the body comes into a healthy equilibrium.

A colleague of mine, Rhonda, once walked around the corner

of her house in the mountainous desert region of southern California to see why her dog was barking. What awaited her was a mountain lion emerging from her garage.

Her heart started pounding, her blood pressure elevated, her gut instinctively froze her in place, and she screamed. The mountain lion, probably as startled as Rhonda, took off running and jumped the fence.

As she watched it disappear over the fence, her gut relaxed and her heart slowed down as her system began to return to normal. She realized she was no longer in danger. Rhonda came out of her frozen state as she picked up her dog and walked back into her house to call her neighbor. Her breathing had normalized completely by the time she picked up the phone.

This area of the prefrontal cortex worked with her body signals to come back to equilibrium relatively quickly. As a desert rancher, Rhonda had survived many different types of scenarios like this, so her body had a resilience that helped her nervous system return to normal quickly. This allowed her to be ready for whatever life was going to bring next — a vital survival skill in this part of the country!

Brain Idioms

Get your head on straight.
She's headstrong.
It was a head-spinning experience.
I'm going out of my mind.
I'm losing my mind.
I can't think straight.
I'm a feather brain.
She's a lame brain.
They are my brain trust.
He's brain-dead.
He has sports on the brain.
I was blindsided.
My brain is sweating.
It was a lightbulb moment.
My head is in the game.
He's in a brain fog.
She's an egghead.
Those kids are rattle-brained.
I'm wracking my brain to understand.
I need more brain power.
The show was highbrow.
He's all brawn, no brain.
He's a smarty-pants.
That's brain food.
My higher brain is resting.
My lower brain just hijacked me.

Healthy Communication

When we perceive other people's signals, resonate with those signals, and respond back in ways that allow us to connect more deeply with them, life feels good. Nurturing connection is a foundational need for health and well-being. When this area is not working well, signals get mixed up or misinterpreted, and disconnection and pain can be the outcome.

One of my clients, Joe, was at a party, and he looked across the room and saw Melissa smiling at him. His heart skipped a beat as he thought about approaching her. The warmth in her smile, which touched his heart, was just the signal he needed to come and speak to her. He walked across the room and introduced himself. His brain had picked up the signal from his heart, interpreted it, and he took action.

Joe and Melissa had a spirited conversation. Joe's heart was really on fire with her intelligent wit and beauty. Melissa seemed equally smitten. As they talked, Joe made a political comment that caused Melissa to drop her smile. Although she did not walk away, Melissa was distinctly cooler in her words and manner thereafter. Joe's heart sank as he perceived these signals and recognized that he had made a big mistake. His heart was accurately picking up the signals from Melissa, and his brain's perception of these signals allowed a deeper communication than words alone.

All of us as human beings are in this kind of deeper communication in every moment of our lives. It is so important that our social engagement systems be working well in order for our lives to feel connected to those that matter most to us.

Emotional Balance

The triage office of the prefrontal cortex modulates a healthy balance point between too much emotional arousal and too little — in other words, to calm or inhibit excessive emotions and allow healthy emotions to arise and inform us of whatever information they have to offer.

My colleague Peter had to give a speech at his brother's wedding. When he stood up, his fear of public speaking overtook him. His heart was racing, and he could not speak. He dropped his attention down into his legs and feet to ground himself; as he settled further into his bones, his thoughts cleared. With this, he recognized that his body's response was not really appropriate to the situation — he was not actually in danger.

Peter slowed his breathing and felt the gratitude and love he had for his brother. Looking out on the faces of family and friends, he realized that everyone in the room wished him well. His heart rate slowed as the fear subsided, and Peter delivered his speech and received a standing ovation.

Here we can see how the prefrontal cortex area and our body wisdom areas are in partnership to help modulate emotions that would otherwise paralyze us.

As a public speaker myself for over thirty years, I know that when I am speaking and my emotions (usually tears) start to rise because of a story I am sharing, if I simply remember to drop my awareness downward and inward in my body, it steadies me and allows for the point to be delivered powerfully yet calmly.

Response Flexibility

The ability to pause before responding — as we weigh our options and choose the most appropriate response — is vital for *not* being hijacked by the emotional arousal centers in the brain.

Recently, a good friend, Mary, was sitting in her car at a red light. She jumped in her seat, startled, when the person behind her began honking his horn.

Her first response was irritation. She wanted to yell at him, "The light is still red — can't you see that?" Then she felt shame about that response, thinking that maybe the man needed to get through for some reason. Perhaps she was in the way. Her midsection felt contracted, and it tightened more by the minute.

Mary felt herself instinctively move her foot to the gas pedal. But she paused and reassessed the situation. Finally, she realized that the man was honking at a friend walking down the sidewalk.

The capacity human beings have to modulate emotional responses is vast, when we pause and take the time to see the bigger picture.

Insight

The ability to connect the past with the present moment and the anticipated future provides us with the perspective to make wise choices.

Any conscious healing requires bringing our unprocessed past memories to light in order to understand them and loosen the grip of the emotional charge they may still hold for us.

Insight helps us see how our past and future affect who we are right now. When we cultivate insight, it awakens us to the traits we have that we would like to broaden or change in some way.

Insight gives us the capacity to become active and empowered in understanding the inner stories or personal narratives that may have previously driven our actions and personality unconsciously.

In chapter 3, I describe Tony, the overcaring nurse practitioner; his unconscious mandate or inner narrative about taking care of others literally drove him to a heart attack. His example might very well be the natural consequence of a disconnection between his body's wisdom — which told him to slow down and rest — and the insight capacity in this area of the brain, which normally would receive the body's signals and act upon them in a way that would lead to health, not a heart attack.

I recently interviewed a woman who is a top manager in a healthcare organization. After a serious health scare, she got the message from her body and has reconnected her insight capacities to the body signals she receives daily.

Now, when she feels that heavy, tired sensation that used to be the precursor to her health breakdown, she rests — no excuses. She is also changing her lifestyle to include more yoga and meditation.

As this occurs, she is literally integrating her past experiences into her present-moment sensations and is now able to see and live into a much healthier future.

Empathy

Empathy describes the way we understand another's point of view, which may include the ability to feel a similar sensation or emotion or have an image of their experience in our own mind.

This area of the brain registers the heartfelt connections and other body senses that naturally arise when we are in another person's presence and recognize their current feeling state or broader life situation.

Recently, a dear friend of mine died suddenly, and the next day happened to be his wife's birthday. How do you celebrate your birthday and grieve the loss of your beloved all in one twenty-four-hour period? My empathy for her situation was great. My heart went out to her, and I reached out to let her know she was not alone.

I speak to this in chapter 1. When we do not know how to manage our empathy, it is not going to feel like an asset. When we feel bombarded by what others are feeling due to our own sensitivity, the tendency is to turn our empathy off — either by blocking the incoming body signals or by numbing out what this area of the brain is telling us.

Whether we block or numb empathy, we are the poorer for it because it also locks us out of the richness of the deep connection possibilities that life holds. These connections can help us feed and repair painful past memories of disconnection and loneliness.

Recently, during a craniosacral class demonstration, the woman I was treating, Martha, described a painful disconnection from her parents. They fought endlessly, leaving her feeling alone and abandoned by the age of three.

As she described this, Martha welled up with tears. Much of the audience was touched by the poignancy of her experience. Through the session, Martha resolved and released her limiting belief of continual and unending abandonment. The session ended with her feeling full and energized, even joyful.

After the demo, an older man said that he, too, had felt tears welling up as she described her experience. He shared that he also had a history of deep and painful disconnection in his early childhood. He wanted to know how he could be a therapist and hold space for this level of anguish without drowning in his own pain?

In my experience, this is not an uncommon dilemma. I gently helped him settle back and ground himself. When he was able to embody at that level, his entire countenance changed.

His face relaxed, and he realized not only could he hold his own pain, but he could be in the presence of another's pain without becoming overwhelmed. In that moment, he was also able to feel the joy-filled place Martha experienced by the end of the session.

When our inner emotional world is in chaos or pain, the tendency is to clamp down and try to control or contain it. This response blocks empathy and keeps us from moving forward in life.

The healthy alternative is integration of our emotional world, bringing empathy onboard as an asset instead of a liability.

Fear Modulation

We have the capacity to mediate fear that would normally cripple us. GABA is an inhibitory peptide that quiets the overfiring hypervigilance that comes with a fear response.

When we can purposefully, mindfully modulate our fear, as Peter did above in the wedding speech for his brother, research shows that the prefrontal cortex grows connecting fibers down into the trauma-registering areas of the brain and provides them with calming GABA.[3]

Deep core embodiment practices, like the ones suggested in this book, calm anxiety and fear by creating integrative connections to this area of the brain.

My experience has been that when people in my trainings utilize these skills, their fear and anxiety levels drop significantly. Their capacity to stay fully functional and effective in stressful situations steadily rises. In fact, this is one of the most commonly reported consequences when these practices are used consistently.

Accessing Intuition

Intuition comes from our inner felt senses, including our gut hunches, our heart's wisdom, our bone-deep clarity, and any other signals our body can offer in its infinite wisdom. Combined with any memories or brain knowing, as well as signals we are picking up from the unseen world and environment around us, this gives us access to perceptions we can trust.

Intuition can show up in many ways. We may have a fleeting thought about someone, and they call moments later. We could feel a wave of sorrow and learn later that a good friend died at the exact moment we felt the sadness.

When these areas are all connected and integrated, this intuitive sense actually begins to feel downright ordinary, meaning that it happens so frequently that you stop questioning it and recognize it as a normal process.

Morality

Our inner moral compass is registered in the prefrontal cortex when our entire system is integrated. In my experience, it works in concert with the wisdom areas of the body, especially the clarity and steadiness of the bones and the deep inspiration and compassion of the heart.

When we have embodied the wisdom areas, and the morality area of the brain is operational, we have a natural capacity to imagine what fulfills the larger social good. This morality does not depend on whether someone is watching us. It comes from within. It enables us to imagine and take action that reflects our inner sense of moral integrity.

Damaged individuals whose middle prefrontal cortexes have been taken off-line by trauma can lose this capacity for moral thinking and action.

I saw this firsthand in the life of my late brother, who sustained two severe head traumas to this exact area of his brain before the age of ten.

The first happened around the age of seven when he ran full-steam into an iron pole on the playground. That injury left him at home for days with a headache as he slowly recovered enough to return to school.

The second incident happened the following year, when he walked up behind me as I was swinging a baseball bat while warming up for a game. This was no light tap to his forehead. I felt horrible as I watched the huge goose egg rise in the middle of his forehead.

As he grew into adolescence, my brother became more and more secretive, and he eventually committed suicide at the age of forty-two, after leading a life of crime that only his inner circle knew about.

When we were both in our twenties, I asked him why he didn't pursue medical school, since he had been pre-med in college.

He looked at me, and in a moment of blunt honesty, which was quite rare for him, he confided that he did not want to help people the way I did. He just didn't care. He was not saying it meanly. He was just being honest.

That inner sense of morality and empathy was off-line in his system, and the actions he took across the next two decades until his death reflected this fact.

Integration

Responsible for overall integration throughout our system, the prefrontal cortex receives input from the body, and it connects directly with the other cortex layers, the limbic area of the brain, and the brain stem.

It is responsible for creating social integration, bodily integration, limbic integration, and brain-stem integration. All of these important areas come together in the triage office of the prefrontal cortex of the brain.

There are other areas of the brain that register body sensations and processes — the insula, the thalamus, the pituitary and hypothalamus, and many more, which are being uncovered and discovered every day.[4] What we know is that there are many interconnections between the structures in the brain and our body wisdom, which support the practices described in this book.

As you can see, it is important to include the brain in our team of body wisdom areas.

However, it is not the boss it was thought to be for so long. The top-down model is outdated. A model that reflects the partnership of the body wisdom and all the areas of the brain is gaining acceptance. Much of what happens is actually coming from the bottom up, and we need to recognize this fact and work with a new integrated body wisdom model so we can experience our full potential. This chapter's exploration will help you do just that; to download the audio, go to www.healingfromthecore.com, click on the Reclaiming Your Body Download link, and enter the password *presence*.

EXPLORATION

Integrated Body Wisdom Exploration

The following practice will help you to better navigate from your unique inner landscape by awakening your awareness in some of the key wisdom areas of your body and listening to what they have to share with you.

Feel free to do Explorations 1 (pages 55–59) and 2 (pages 59–66) prior to this exploration for a deeper experience. Also remember that Exploration 3 (pages 66–79) is designed to be used whenever you hit a roadblock or some kind of resistance in your Core Embodiment Process — so if, as you are exploring each of the different wisdom areas, you uncover some resistance, that would be an indicator to use Exploration 3 (but certainly not to give up and tell yourself the process simply does not work or does not work for you).

Inner Awareness

We begin by simply taking a baseline of your inner awareness, without trying to change anything. To do this, allow your feet to rest fully on the floor, eyes closed or semiclosed. As you settle in, following your breath, be curious about the temperature of the air as it enters your nostrils and fills your lungs.

Notice the rise and fall of your chest and back as you breathe normally.

Wisdom of the Heart

Allow your awareness to travel to the area of your heart, dropping your attention inside, as deeply as is comfortable at this time. What sensations show up here? Does it feel warm or cool? Does it feel like a particular color? Is there a hum or a pulse?

The heart is well known as the home of our caring, compassion, and love. Travel to an even more profound level, and the heart is the wisdom keeper of our deepest inspirations, keeping our inner fire burning.

What is it that inspires you most in your life right now? What lights up your days and energizes you? Feel where it resides in your heart. What is the sensation of it? What images arise?

You might be inspired by a project you're involved with, or something in your own healing process, or raising a family, or creating something new and exciting.

Whatever it is, allow yourself to notice what it feels like in your heart as you breathe into and acknowledge this inspiration in your life right now.

Wisdom of the Gut

Next, allow your awareness to drop down under your heart into your belly-gut area, noticing how this wisdom area is informing whatever inspiration lives in your heart. Does it feel connected to your heart? Is the connection weak or strong?

As your attention rests there, notice whether your gut is telling you how right this inspiration is for you, or perhaps how it needs to be changed in order to bring it to fruition.

If there's something that's a little off about how you are experiencing your inspiration, that instinctual gut feeling will inform you of it. Register what your gut is saying to you right now. Listen to it.

What we are looking for here is a natural alignment and full connection between your gut knowing and what inspires you. If there's something that isn't quite right yet, you can make an adjustment until it does sit right between your instinctual wisdom and what lights your inner fire.

The gut's wisdom offers important feedback moment to moment. This information is vital to listen to in order to take action on *only* those things that are truly right for you at this time.

Wisdom of the Pelvis

Next, allow your awareness to drop down into your pelvis, into the engine of your body. This includes your pelvic floor and reproductive system, as well as your sacrum and coccyx.

Does it feel open and connected to your gut and heart? What sensations do you feel here?

The questions answered by this wisdom area are, "Am I willing to put my power behind this deep inspiration in my heart? Do I *have* the power to support what it needs?"

Just notice what your pelvis says and whether you feel as though you *can* support this project, this inspiration, from this natural well of energy — rather than your will. This area will also inform you if the strength is or is not there at this time.

It may signal you that you need to regroup or slow down what you are doing. This is quite helpful if you are an optimistic dreamer who needs the energy "reality check" that the pelvis has for you.

It may give you a full "go ahead" signal, which can ignite your dreams and inspirations and help you take the next step to manifesting them.

Wisdom of the Legs and Feet

Sometimes there are many sides to an issue, and layers of complexity to deal with in any given idea, quest, or inspiration — perplexing problems to be solved, barriers to be met and dissolved. When this occurs, as is often the case in our lives, the wisdom of the legs and feet are needed.

If you can take an actual walk at this point, that is ideal.

If not, imagine yourself taking a walk with this issue, dropping down into your legs and on down into your feet, breathing and stimulating the desire to move forward on this deep inspiration. Our legs and feet can help us with integrating the whole process.

In your mind's eye, take this walk somewhere that's beautiful for you so that your attention is on the scenery, and you can let everything "digest" without thinking about it.

Imagine yourself walking at a comfortable pace, swinging your arms, your heart pumping. As this occurs, effortlessly it metabolizes or digests the issue you are mulling over. This cross-body movement integrates the right and left hemispheres of your brain as well as moving it throughout the rest of your system.

When you're ready, let your walk come to an end and notice what new information or answers appear in your consciousness.

Wisdom of the Bones

Next, allow your awareness to drop into your bones, deep into your innermost recesses — those sturdy, steady parts of who you are. Your bones are your densest, strongest connective tissue, and most of them exist deep in the core of your body. They form the structure upon which everything else rests.

Feeling your spine, your pelvic bones, or your legs and feet. Pick whichever of these areas feel easy to sink into in this moment, and rest there with your attention deep inside of you.

Remember, our bones are like sponges with air spaces, and allow yourself to breathe into the air spaces of your bones...with each breath, dropping deeper into your bones.

Take a few minutes now to sit in silence with your awareness deep inside.

[Pause]

Notice the clarity that comes as the mud of your life's activities settles, and you sit deeper in the calmness your bones naturally provide. Take as long as you need to feel the steadying, clear sense that this wisdom area provides. Notice the deep informing coming from your bones.

[Pause]

Wisdom of Integrated Body Awareness

When you have rested in your bones long enough, allow your awareness to begin to expand from your bones out into all the rest of your body, infusing it with a clear sense of direction and steadiness. From deep inside, like a gentle mist, expanding from the inner temple of your bones, let all the cells of your body be drenched in this wisdom.

Allow this expansion to include your head, your brain. Let the wisdom of your heart, gut, pelvis, legs and feet, and bones share information with the great creator and map maker in your brain, so that you're able to visualize what you want clearly, strategize and make wise plans, and see what step comes next. Let this process unfold, coming to you easily and naturally.

When you're ready, allow your awareness to return to the outer world. You may want to take out your journal and make some notes about what you saw and felt and heard from these deep wisdom areas of your body, so you can follow through in your life.

And enjoy!

11

Living in All Our Cells

Life Is Waiting for You

People say that what we're all seeking is a meaning for life.
I don't think that's what we're really seeking. I think that
what we're seeking is an experience of being alive,
so that our life experiences on the purely physical plane
will have resonances with our own innermost being and reality,
so that we actually feel the rapture of being alive.

— JOSEPH CAMPBELL

In the fall of 1983, when I attended my first CranioSacral Therapy (CST) class with Dr. John Upledger, my body's signals started full-out yelling at me. At the time of that first class, I lived with daily chronic pain from a car accident in 1980 (not to mention the remnants of neck issues from 1971), and my body's wisdom somehow recognized that this system of healing held the key to freedom from my pain.

On the last day of class, as I watched Dr. Upledger do this full-body release demonstration, every remaining pain-ridden cell in my body started aching for that healing attention. It went from a low background noise to full-blown pain, as though to say to him, "Over here!" I could not ignore what I felt. It was so palpable it could not be missed.

I had no explanation for how my body knew. Although I may not have explained it this way at the time, I know now that my heart felt deeply inspired, and my gut knew this work was the path to my healing. I knew that I was in the presence of something that could help me.

This is what happens for me when a path opens that I am meant to take. I know that I am not the only one to experience this. I imagine as you are reading this paragraph you may be feeling something in your body that is registering what I am saying, perhaps taking this opportunity to inform you of something you had not noticed until now. If this is occurring for you, please take a moment and acknowledge it.

In the early 1980s, there was not a lot of understanding, much less research, to back up what I was learning and experiencing. I just knew it was right for me. When I finally became one of the initial instructors of CST in 1986, we were just a small group from many disciplines who taught the work with Dr. Upledger.

We were all very well trained, but to a certain degree, we operated on faith in him because, beyond his textbooks, the left-brain understanding and research just was not there yet. And while he loved and appreciated us, he was not the kind of guy who would sit down with us and hash out the details that were still not clear in our heads. Questions like, how do you logically explain cellular intelligence, tissue memory, and bodily wisdom?

What kept us all going were the results, the clinical outcomes we were experiencing with our clients and students — the woman whose sense of smell returned after twenty years from a short CST demo that released her hard palate and ethmoid bone; the male student whose vision cleared after a particularly big release of his sphenoid in a demo; the client whose bite returned to normal in three CST sessions after years of struggle with dental appliances; the back surgery client whose pain was worse after surgery but felt it dissolve in one CST treatment on his dural tube; and the teenage lacrosse player whose three days of head pain dissolved after one treatment.

Then there was my own experience. I began getting CST treatments soon after that initial class, and layer by layer the pain released. In 1987, in an intensive advanced training, the last of my pain disappeared. That was it for me. Dr. Upledger always talked about how the intelligence of our cells is infinite and powerful, but having the experience come home to my own body made it irrefutable.

I didn't care what anyone else said. I knew CST was effective for me, and I knew beyond a shadow of a doubt that my cells held wisdom that was just waiting to be heard. I had actual personal corroboration — the felt sense in my own body. I began listening more closely to all parts of my body. Using my body's wisdom — listening to and being present in my heart, my gut, my pelvis, and my bones for healing and guidance. I developed Healing from the Core (HFC) to share this knowledge and experience with others.

The Experience of Full-Body Presence

As I complete this book, I am in residence at the Esalen Institute in Big Sur, California, and the exquisiteness of life awakens and deepens in me as I write, despite my looming deadline.

There are moments when I am walking — present in my legs and feet — from my little yurt to the lodge, up and down the steep hills and through the dirt path of the garden, and the parade of scents fills my nostrils. I realize that life is completely full of bursts of joyous experience, which I feel throughout my body but most strongly in my heart.

As I leave my yurt, I am first touched by the smell of the eucalyptus trees overhead, followed soon by the rosemary bushes and then wild fennel. Around the curve is the intoxicating scent of the jasmine vines growing over the laundry-building wall, followed by the roses and the sweet peas and something else that my body loves but cannot identify. This simple walk fills my soul. I enter the lodge for meals with a smile on my face.

And what I am describing is just from my sense of smell!

I can easily expand this experience. There is the tingling coolness on my skin upon crossing the narrow wooden footbridge over the stream of clean, living water — tumbling over rocks and trees on its way to the ocean. In this part of my walk, my ears also get fed — no, drenched — in the soft, strong sounds of this clear, sparkling movement of the water. It demands my attention. It reminds me of the fluid aliveness of my pelvis and my passion for my life. I listen and am filled with the sounds of living, moving water.

Then there is the visual scene, which is beyond anything I have known anywhere else. Hundreds of feet above the ocean, some days are gray and mysterious, hidden by the foggy marine layer; some days are sparkling and dancing with white caps. The vastness of this vista is…majestic and magical. The fingers of fog rolling in, the sunsets each night, the moment when the sun first breaks through in the morning and lights up the treetops — can you see it? I am grateful for my mind, my brain, which allows me to perceive and put into words the beauty of this magical place.

When I turn my eyes to the land, everywhere I look there is color and texture and life. The gardens and grounds are tended with love and are beautiful without looking manicured. There is a "high-definition" visual beauty even in the wildness here, perhaps because of the combination of ocean air and clear sunlight.

I share all of this not to celebrate Esalen in particular, but to emphasize that this *direct experience* of life can happen *anywhere* when you are open to it and fully present in your body in the moment.

This is how we can live when we are awakened: mind, body,

and spirit. This is what Joseph Campbell was talking about in this chapter's epigraph when he said: "I think that what we're seeking is an experience of being alive, so that our life experiences on the purely physical plane will have resonances with our own innermost being and reality, so that we actually feel the rapture of being alive."[1]

I have had this quote on a shelf in my office for over four decades. It called to my inner body wisdom then, before I had any clear understanding of it, and it still speaks to me today.

I am so grateful for my healing. I am no longer the little girl traumatized by too early an entry to kindergarten, the churchgoer with no lower-body presence, or the teenager in chronic shock from a physical attack. I have healed by listening to the wisdom of my body.

The *rapture of being alive* is not something we accomplish, organize, will ourselves into, or experience all the time, yet with full-body presence we can open to it, allow it, and be with it.

Body wisdom can help you heal from trauma and make it possible to awaken to all the cells of your body with more frequency and more depth.

We are not just our body, and yet our bodies are the physical foundation of our experience of being alive, in this incredible universe of streaming energy, which can nourish us, moment to moment, day to day, week in and week out, if only we engage with curiosity, awareness, and trust.

12

Opening to Life Intentionally

Action Steps for Twenty-Eight Days

A t the end of chapter 10, I mention the concept of living from our integrated body wisdom — one that informs us and grows as we live our lives from within the exquisite navigational system of our body.

Are we more than just our body? Of course. And yet our integrated body wisdom is truly the missing link for most people today. It is the foundation for so much else.

So we come back to the question:

What is your current relationship with your body?

Take a moment now and retake the "Body Intelligence Quiz" in chapter 1 (pages 9–11).

Are any of your answers different this time?

Is your inner landscape starting to send signals that you can recognize?

Remember, the body operates optimally by consensus. Every cell, every part of who we are, is meant to be in good relationship with all the others. Our conscious awareness is meant to be in consensual partnership with our body. This means befriending our whole body. Any part left out of this conversation can be problematic.

In this chapter, I present four weeks of practices to systematically support your inner growth. This provides a simple structured process for diving into your inner landscape more deeply. Once you have read them through, find time to commit to them and begin!

A Practical Tool to Help — Journaling

When following these practices, I suggest journaling or somehow recording what shows up as you go. This tool is invaluable.

I am often asked: Why journal? What's in it for me?

Journaling offers a window to your inner workings, showing you things you may not have even realized were there until the words hit the page.

What's more, research has shown that the process of simply identifying, acknowledging, and writing about your experiences lowers stress hormones, assists in brain integration, and can initiate the healing process.

Journaling is an opportunity for calm awareness. It is one of the many practices that help us filter out the chatter in our minds and listen to the quiet voice within.

As you read the questions and prompts below, write down as much of your experience as you can remember — write as fast as you can.

Don't worry about spelling or punctuation. Just let the words flow out onto the page. If you are inspired to draw or add color, do it. Do whatever it takes to record the experience as fully as possible for you.

Journaling can lead to discovery. Respect your own process as you write. You may want to take a break and come back a few minutes later to read your words with fresh eyes.

Gather your journal or prepare something to record your words, thoughts, images, and sensations as you do the following exploration and answer the following questions.

Week One

For the first week, I suggest that you make a daily practice of doing Exploration 1: Opening Awareness (see pages 55–59), and journaling whatever arises. In addition, journal your answers to the three questions below. This will thoroughly introduce you to your inner landscape.

As you do, remember the attributes of curiosity, awareness, and trust, which I mention in chapter 4. Everything that arises is simply information. Cultivate curiosity about what shows up. Your experience is expanding your awareness day by day.

Lastly, trust what you get. Please do not let your judgmental mind hijack the bus of your growing awareness. Trust that your inner landscape has valuable information — what I call "deep informing" — when you allow it to come forward unimpeded.

Here is a series of questions (in italics) to ask yourself as you listen to the audio exploration. They encourage you to dive deeper to assess where you are now in order to map out how to proceed optimally. Ask yourself:

What parts of my body do I like?

These areas are where you feel most comfortable and present, where it is easiest to sense what it feels like on a good day.

What parts do I dislike?

These areas may feel like they are pushing you away, or they may feel painful or tight or be holding tension. They may feel numb or distant, as though they are not connected to the rest of you.

What parts do I need onboard that are not currently on my team?

These parts may directly overlap with what you dislike or shy away from about your body. Then again, some surprises may show up. Listen and be open to discovery.

These places may be in or around important wisdom areas.

For example, you might become aware that your throat is quite tight, causing you to go mute when you want to speak from the true voice of your heart.

Or you may not be able to feel much of anything, sensation-wise, in your pelvis.

Or there may be a tight, achy sensation in your gut that keeps you from being able to accurately register the current-moment instinctual hits that you need in order to feel safe without being hypervigilant.

As you journal the answers to these questions, you may find that other thoughts, images, and hits arise. Feel free to write or draw them as well.

Week Two

For week two, utilize Exploration 2: The Core Embodiment Process (see pages 59–66) on a daily basis. This allows you to practice replenishing your inner energy reservoir — the container of your body. Experiment with what time of day is best and where you like to practice this exploration.

Some enjoy starting their day with it, while others like to end their day and drift off to a good night's sleep with it. Others like to close their office door at lunchtime and take a break with it.

This practice is the cornerstone for core embodiment. It deepens and evolves with time, allowing you to feel more comfortable inside your own skin.

Once again, everything that arises is simply information. Cultivate a curiosity about what shows up. Be open to discovering new sensations. The exploration will awaken and expand your awareness day by day.

As always, trust what you get. Please do not judge your experience. And journal to reflect on the valuable information that arises.

Week Three

With two weeks of daily practice, you will have grown a better sense of the container of who you are, feeling more and more present within your body and the energy field that flows through it and around it.

By now you are also no doubt noticing the places where you feel disconnected, distant, in pain, tight, or uncomfortable. These may be the places that had a more difficult time soaking up nourishing and nurturing sensations as you did your Core Embodiment Process each day. These may be new places that are showing up in surprising ways as you awaken to new inner awareness.

Now you are ready for Exploration 3: Healing the Internal Resistance to Life (see pages 66–79). Once again, find a time that works for you. Then listen to the exploration daily for the week, or as often as possible, and experience what comes up for healing and integration.

Journal your experience. Draw or paint your experience. Take your time. Slow down the process if necessary. But stay the course. This exploration provides powerful and yet gentle tools for deeper healing and integration.

In dealing with life's smaller issues, you may find that the "aha" moment comes in one round of the practice. With other issues, it may be a week of working with it repeatedly.

If you have a long-held pocket of trauma, you may have to return to it daily as the layers of it peel away and dissolve in a manner that you can integrate. Take it at your own pace.

You may find that, like me with my serious chronic pain, it takes years of releasing and healing. However, if you are going in a direction that is ultimately healing and life-enhancing, you will feel better and better as each layer lets go. The healing process also becomes easier and easier. And life gets richer and richer.

Again, stay the course — you are cultivating a new relationship with your body and with your mind and spirit as well.

Be patient and trust that your cellular intelligence is engaging
with you. Trust that your inner wisdom knows what direction and
at what pace your healing should unfold.

You are doing your part by showing up, committing to listening, engaging with openness and curiosity, and responding to the
deep informing that arises from within you.

Be kind to yourself in this process. Love yourself as deeply as
you can right now. It is this love — this all-encompassing deep
caring — that will carry you home to yourself.

Week Four

This week is about reaping the benefits of the healing processes
you have been practicing for three weeks.

Now set aside the time to have an even more intimate conversation with your inner landscape.

Every day, practice the Integrated Body Wisdom Exploration
(see pages 166–70), and journal and listen to the deep informing
that shows up — whether through feelings, images, words, colors,
or textures — and let it all in.

By using this Integrated Body Wisdom Exploration every
day, you are offering exponentially more deep informing and wisdom to every decision in your life. Openness to discovery brings
magical synchronicities, infinite possibilities, and creativity in all
areas of your life.

Remember, this work is about *experiencing* life. It's about
having more joyful moments and healthier connections, while
being able to hold those areas within where pain still exists with
love and tenderness for healing.

Though I have described the structure that offers you this
experience, the choice is yours. Will you take it?

Acknowledgments

Once again, it has taken a village to complete this book. As my work with touch that heals, embodiment, and trauma resolution has matured in the last decade, this book was forming inside of me. There have been a number of dear and loving friends and colleagues who have contributed with their own stories, by working alongside me, or by inspiring me. I hope I can remember and honor everyone who has been a part of this incredible process.

My first thanks must go to Chery Owens, who has been my steady editor throughout this book. Then Kim Falone and Robyn Scherr, who contributed some key points at the beginning and end of it all. Then to Rachel Abrams, who collaborated with me on the BQ assessment for both our books, and her husband, my wonderful literary agent, Doug Abrams.

Next are my HFC instructors for steadily believing in the work we are pioneering together, as well as my HFC presenter and practitioner staff, who have been in the trenches with me as I led the workshops where these ideas were born and tested.

The rest of the village — who were my readers or donated their time brainstorming or editing — get my next wave of gratitude. This includes Debbie Behnfield, Valerie Bowman, Dorie

Christman, Kelly Dorfman, Erica Eickhoff, Patrice Ficken, Chris Hendricks, Kate Mackinnon, and Joel Ying.

I am sure there are others I am forgetting. It has been years' worth of asking for and receiving help from my entire village. Thank you all from the bottom of my heart.

I must also acknowledge Michael Kern for seeing me clearly and bringing me together with Dan Siegel, Stephen Porges, Peter Levine, and Bessel van der Kolk, who then graciously allowed me into their inner circle to learn and grow with them — all generous men.

Susan Harper and the late Emilie Conrad have been my largest inspiration and mentors in the embodiment arena — both generous women dedicated to exploring the edge of who we are as human beings, who taught me not to be afraid on that edge myself.

The Upledger Institute's entire staff, especially John Matthew Upledger, have been an immense support for my trainings and the work this book is based upon. The late Dr. John Upledger and CranioSacral Therapy are the foundation this book rests upon — I am immensely grateful for all I have received there.

The Esalen Institute's magical space and staff have supported my work on so many levels, not the least of which was giving me the time and space to write the last chapters of this book in September 2016. Thank you all!

I could not have completed this book without my dedicated Healing from the Core office team, starting with Christy Allison, Lynn Foley, Sharon Desjarlais, and Elizabeth Charles — all generous women with their time, writing gifts, and other efforts on my behalf.

Then the next wave of gratitude goes out to all the students and clients whose experiences have enriched my life and this book. Your stories have taught me valuable lessons that were passed forward here.

Finally, the biggest wave of gratitude goes out to my family members, who have supported and encouraged me throughout this entire process — my husband, Carlos; my daughter, Alieza; my son, Aren; my sister, Debbie; and my mom, Mary Jane, to whom I dedicated this book. You all have supported me in ways large and small that made this book possible.

I love you all.

Notes

Chapter 1. The Answers Lie Within: The Journey Begins

1. Bessel van der Kolk, *The Body Keeps the Score: Brain, Mind, and Body in the Healing of Trauma* (New York: Viking Penguin, 2014).
2. Peter Levine, *In an Unspoken Voice* (Lyons, CO: ERGOS Institute Press, 2010), 37.
3. Stephen W. Porges, *The Polyvagal Theory: Neurophysiological Foundations of Emotions, Attachment, Communication, and Self-Regulation* (New York: W.W. Norton & Company, 2011).
4. Porges, *Polyvagal Theory*.
5. Levine, *In an Unspoken Voice*.
6. Judson Brewer, "A Simple Way to Break a Bad Habit," TEDMED Talk, November 2015, http://www.ted.com/talks/judson_brewer_a_simple_way _to_break_a_bad_habit. This talk is based on Judson Brewer and Lori Pbert, "Mindfulness: An Emerging Treatment for Smoking and Other Addictions?" *Journal of Family Medicine* 2, no. 4 (September 3, 2015), among other publications.

Chapter 2. The Five Body Myths: Blind Alleys That Throw Us Off Course

1. Peter Levine, *Waking the Tiger: Healing Trauma* (Berkeley, CA: North Atlantic Books, 1997). This book describes the primal response of the

body to trauma and release as one of trembling, as the system moves from frozen back into healthy movement.

2. Porges, *Polyvagal Theory*. Porges looks closely at the power of healthy connection and how it promotes the feeling of safety, which in turn allows healing to occur.

3. Emilie Conrad, *Life on Land: The Story of Continuum, the World-Renowned Self-Discovery and Movement Method* (Berkeley, CA: North Atlantic Books, 2007).

4. Daniel J. Siegel, *The Neurobiology of "We": How Relationships, the Mind, and the Brain Interact to Shape Who We Are*, Sounds True, 2011, compact disc.

5. Research on the enteric nervous system includes Adam Hadhazy, "Think Twice: How the Gut's 'Second Brain' Influences Mood and Well-Being," *Scientific American* (February 12, 2010), www.scientificamerican.com /article/gut-second-brain; Levi Gadye, "The Second Brain: The Science of the Gut Continues to Make Good On Its Promise to Aid in the Understanding and Treatment of Mental Disorders and Beyond," *Berkeley Science Review* (December 30, 2013); and Jay Pashricha, "The Brain-Gut Connection," Johns Hopkins Medicine, www.hopkinsmedicine.org /health/healthy_aging/healthy_body/the-brain-gut-connection.

6. For research into the human capacity to sense and intuit information before the eye can see it, or before it can be sensed in any other way, see Rupert Sheldrake, *The Sense of Being Stared At* (Rochester, VT: Park Street Press, 2013); and Rollin McCraty, *The Science of the Heart: Exploring the Role of the Heart in Human Performance* (Boulder Creek, CA: Heart-Math, 2015).

7. John E. Upledger, *SomatoEmotional Release and Beyond* (Palm Beach Gardens, FL: UI Publishers, 1990).

Chapter 3. The Hallmarks of Optimum Health:
Finding the Path Home

1. Kolk, *The Body Keeps the Score*, 155–68.

2. Centers for Disease Control and Prevention, CDC-Kaiser Permanente Adverse Childhood Experiences (ACE) Study, accessed September 15, 2016, https://www.cdc.gov/violenceprevention/acestudy/about.html.

3. Ibid.; Nadine Burke Harris, "How Childhood Trauma Affects Health

Across a Lifetime," TEDMED Talk, September 2014, https://www.ted
.com/talks/nadine_burke_harris_how_childhood_trauma_affects_health
_across_a_lifetime.

4. Abram Kardiner, "The Traumatic Neuroses of War" (1941), cited in Kolk, *The Body Keeps the Score*, 11.

5. Gabor Maté, *When the Body Says No: Exploring the Stress-Disease Connection* (Hoboken, NJ: John Wiley & Sons, 2003).

6. With his polyvagal theory, Stephen Porges talks in detail about the vagus nerve and how it controls everything from our salivary glands to our rectum when there is a sense of danger or a sense of love and safety. See Porges, *Polyvagal Theory*.

7. Ashley Montagu, *Touching: The Human Significance of the Skin*, 2nd ed. (New York: Harper & Row, 1978).

8. Bessel van der Kolk, "Forward," quoted in Peter A. Levine, *Trauma and Memory: Brain and Body in a Search for the Living Past* (Berkeley, CA: North Atlantic Books, 2015), xv.

Chapter 4. Embodying Fully: Practices to Live By

1. All three explorations in this chapter can also be found in my book *Full Body Presence: Learning to Listen to Your Body's Wisdom* (Novato, CA: New World Library, 2010).

Chapter 5. Your Heart: The Gift of Inspiration

1. See Doc Lew Childre, *The HeartMath Solution: The Institute of Heart-Math's Revolutionary Program for Engaging the Power of the Heart's Intelligence* (New York: HarperCollins, 1999); and Rollin McCraty, *Science of the Heart, Volume 2: Exploring the Role of the Heart in Human Performance* (Boulder Creek, CA: HeartMath, 2015). Much more research is available on HeartMath's website, www.heartmath.com/research (accessed September 30, 2016).

Chapter 6. Your Gut: The Gift of Instinctual Knowing

1. Gavin de Becker, *The Gift of Fear: And Other Survival Signals That Protect Us from Violence* (New York: Dell Publishing, 1997).

2. Emeran Mayer, "The Mysterious Origins of Gut Feelings," TEDx

UCLA, July 2015, http://tedxtalks.ted.com/video/The-mysterious-origins-of-gut-feeling.

3. The prefrontal cortex area of the brain has been found in recent research to act as an inner triage office that takes incoming sensory data and information from the body and uses it to make wiser life choices.

4. For more on Somatic Experiencing, see the books of Peter A. Levine.

5. "Exercise and Depression," Harvard Medical School (Harvard Health Publications, June 2009), accessed September 30, 2016, http://www.health.harvard.edu/mind-and-mood/exercise-and-depression-report-excerpt. See also James A. Levine, "What Are the Risks of Sitting Too Much?" Mayo Clinic, www.mayoclinic.org/healthy-lifestyle/adult-health/expert-answers/sitting/faq-20058005.

6. Brewer, "A Simple Way to Break a Bad Habit."

Chapter 7. Your Pelvis: The Gift of Power

1. Naomi Wolf, *Vagina: Revised and Updated* (New York: HarperCollins, 2013).

2. Ibid., 87–126.

Chapter 8. Your Legs and Feet: The Gift of Movement

1. To learn more about the Brain Gym curriculum, visit www.braingym.org.

2. "Exercise and Depression," Harvard Medical School.

3. Gregg Braden, *Resilience from the Heart: The Power to Thrive in Life's Extremes* (New York: Hay House, 2015).

4. M. Oppezzo and D. L. Schwartz, "Give Your Ideas Some Legs: The Positive Effect of Walking on Creative Thinking," *Journal of Experimental Psychology: Learning, Memory and Cognition* 40, no. 4 (July 2014), DOI: 10.1037/a0036577.

Chapter 10. Your Brain: The Gifts of an Integrated System

1. The anatomy and function of the prefrontal cortex is thoroughly discussed in the following: Siegel, *The Neurobiology of "We"*; Richard J. Davidson and Sharon Begley, *The Emotional Life of Your Brain* (New York: Penguin Group, 2013); and Richard J. Davidson, *Mind: A Journey to the Heart of Being Human* (New York: W.W. Norton, 2016).

2. The following information is drawn from the work of Dr. Dan Siegel, Richard Davidson, and Sharon Begley; see note 1, above.

3. Siegel, *The Neurobiology of "We."*

4. See Davidson, *Mind*; Robert Ornstein, *The Right Mind: A Cutting Edge Picture of How the Two Sides of the Brain Work* (Orlando, FL: Harcourt Brace & Co., 1997); Robert M. Sapolsky, *Why Zebras Don't Get Ulcers* (New York: Holt Paperbacks, 2004); and Les Fehmi and Jim Robbins, *The Open-Focus Brain: Harnessing the Power of Attention to Heal Mind and Body* (Boston, MA: Trumpeter Books, 2007).

Chapter 11. Living in All Our Cells: Life Is Waiting for You

1. Joseph Campbell, *The Power of Myth* (New York: Anchor Books, 1991).

Resources

Reclaiming Your Body is full of resources and ideas that can be manifest. The notes list the books, TED Talks, and research that have informed what is written here. Also, there are many more resources on our website to help you expand and grow. Please visit www.healingfromthecore.com.

I encourage you to sign up for our online newsletter — as well as my blog, "Presence Matters" — to learn about new and exciting resources as they become available. Or attend a Full Body Presence class and experience this work in a safe, supportive group.

It is up to us to choose to go for it, and enjoy!

To write to me about your experiences with this book, visit the websites above or contact:

Healing from the Core Media
PO Box 2534
Reston, VA 20195-2534
office@healingfromthecore.com

Index

About the Author

Suzanne Scurlock-Durana, CMT, CST-D, is one of the world's leading authorities on conscious awareness and its transformational impact on the healing process. For more than thirty years she has empowered people with practical tools that enable them to experience joy in each moment without burning out. These skills help improve every aspect of their lives, from their health and well-being to their relationships, their careers, their creativity, even the growth of their businesses.

After decades of perfecting her methods of awakening the body's innate wisdom, Suzanne created the comprehensive Healing from the Core training curriculum in 1994. Today it includes a robust selection of international workshops, webinars, speaking engagements, and audio programs.

One of the original instructors who was personally mentored by the late Dr. John E. Upledger, Suzanne also continues to teach CranioSacral Therapy and SomatoEmotional Release for the Upledger Institute on nearly every continent. What's more, she collaborated with the late Emilie Conrad for almost two decades. Together they integrated Emilie's Continuum Movement with Suzanne's Full Body Presence to teach other practitioners how to accelerate and deepen the healing process.

Known for her honest, grounded, and nurturing manner, Suzanne is adept at weaving together mind, body, and spirit to create a unique environment that encourages profound healing. She is a sought-after speaker who inspires healthcare providers, coaches, executives, parents, clergy, and others to stay relaxed and energized using her life-changing tools for dissolving stress, pain, overwhelm, and confusion. She also provides ongoing staff development training at the Esalen Institute.

Suzanne has authored hundreds of articles, and thousands of people visit her blog at www.healingfromthecore.com/blog. Plus, she maintains a private practice in Reston, Virginia, where her clients benefit from the innovative techniques she teaches in this book and in her first book, *Full Body Presence: Learning to Listen to Your Body's Wisdom.*

Learn more at www.healingfromthecore.com.

Bright Existence

For Norman & Mary!
with Tremendous
admiration for
your beautiful
Intelligences and
senses of humor
in the halls of
St. Mary's — you
inspire me!
love,
Brenda

Brenda Hillman

Bright Existence

Wesleyan University Press
Published by
University Press of New England
Hanover and London

Wesleyan University Press
Published by University Press of New England, Hanover, NH 03755
© 1993 by Brenda Hillman
All rights reserved
Printed in the United States of America 5 4 3 2 1
CIP *data appear at the end of the book*

1993

For ROBERT HASS

Contents

Acknowledgments

Grateful acknowledgment is made to the following periodicals in which these poems first appeared or will appear, sometimes in different forms:

Agni Review: Steinberg Case (originally "His Shadow")
American Poetry Review: Old Ice, Dark Existence, Black Series, The Servant, December Shadow, January Dawn, March Dawn, Blossoms Appearing, Every Life, A Vigil, First Thought, Adult Joy, Gnostic Heaven, Magdalene, Little Furnace
Antaeus: Dark Matter
The Berkeley Voice: The Rat
The Denver Quarterly: Sorrow of Matter
Epoch: Branch, Scraping, Luminous Textures, and an untitled fragment, (—Why did you tremble . . .)
Equinox: Three untitled fragments, (—Who wounded you . . .), (While I slept you stood . . .), and (—In the cave of the self . . .)
Estero: Vast Fluttering, The Snakeskin
The Nation: Trapped Light
The New Yorker: A Foghorn
The Paris Review: Meridian Plinth, Autumn Moon
Partisan Review: Torn Shadow
Ploughshares: The Spell, Small Spaces
River Styx: Several Errands
The Taos Review: Marshy Area, Useful Shadow, Empty Shadow
Takhum: Holding On
The Threepenny Review: Food, Toll Collector
ZYZZYVA: Mighty Forms, Recycling Center, Spare World

Pushcart Prize XVI reprinted Mighty Forms.

Many thanks to Alex, Fran, James, Joe, John, and Roland.

A Note about the Book

These poems were influenced by my readings in gnosticism, particularly Hans Jonas, to whom I owe a debt, and the old texts in *The Nag Hammadi Library,* which emphasize an inward search for reality, a disjunction between spirit and matter and the soul's individual journey.

In 'the present volume,' the first section finds the soul at dawn, the middle sections move through matter, dailiness and the wounded self, and the final section is a dialogue between love and its shadows. I also owe a debt to the landscapes of West Marin and to Jules Evens for his *Natural History of the Point Reyes Peninsula.*

While I was working on this book, a close friend died, and I wrote *Death Tractates.* It could not be "inserted" into this book, which caused me some difficulty. I now see the two volumes as intimate companions.

Bright Existence

Little Furnace

—Once more the poem woke me up,
the dark poem. I was ready for it;
he was sleeping,

and across the cabin, the small furnace
lit and re-lit itself—the flame a yellow
        "tongue" again, the metal benignly
hard again;

and a thousand insects outside called
        and made me nothing;
moonlight streamed inside as if it had been . . .

I looked around, I thought of the lower wisdom,
spirit held by matter:
        Mary, white as a sand dollar,

and Christ, his sticky halo tilted—
        oh, to get behind it!
The world had been created to comprehend itself

as matter: table, the torn
veils of spiders . . . Even consciousness—
missing my love—

was matter, the metal box of a furnace.
As the obligated flame, so burned my life . . .

What is the meaning of this suffering I asked
and the voice—not Christ but between us—said
you are the meaning.

No no, I replied, That
is the shape, what is the meaning.
You are the meaning, it said—

I. Twelve Dawns

*"A veil exists between the world above and the realms
that are below, and the shadow came into being
beneath the veil, and that shadow became matter."*

(from a Gnostic codex)

Old Ice

The thought that you could even save the light,
that you could stop it from having to be
everywhere at once.

You stood in the ice cream shop
and from the street, in a group
of silly glass trumpets
light came,
and broke into millions of itself, shattered
from the pressure of being mute who knows how long.

There also, leaning against the counter
the child who saw nothing
but the bins of sweet color
separately rimmed with silver.

Behind you, thoughtfully placed by the owners, a photo
of an avalanche, its violence
locked in blue spears . . . The ice moved cruelly, one way only,
and behind the avalanche, and behind
the posts that held it,
the cars went back and forth like mediators.

You who do not exist:
you stared along the edges of the freezer:
froot glistened and clustered.
Suddenly it looked as if one act could be completed,
mounting over and over, even under terrible pressure.
Perhaps the tiny crystals would last forever.

Once it seemed the function of poetry
was to redeem our lives.
But it was not. It was to become
indistinguishable from them.

Dark Existence

—You lay down in your bed
for ten years, and after ten years
you got up. The room was full of weak color

but there was an interesting little hill of rich life
from which all things streamed;

and you saw between
existence and the fringe of your
quotes non-
being on the wall
an active shadow that could not reconcile itself to earth
and was not ironical, that is, not split;

but nothing could be done without some
cooperation between this
shadow and whatever refused it in this world
so you invited it in—

dark existence that comforts and terrifies—
bright existence that could not stay—

Black Series

—Then in the scalloped leaves of the plane tree
a series of short, sharp who's:
a little owl had learned to count.

You lay in your bed as usual not existing
because of the bright edges pressing in.

All at once the black thick o's of the owl
made the very diagram you needed.
Where there had been two
kinds of infinity, now there was one!
The smudged circle around the soul
was the one the gnostics saw around the cosmos,
the mathematical
toy train, the snake eating its tail.

Relieved by the thought that the owl's o's
had changed but not you, that something
could change and not be lost in you,

you asked the voice for more
existence and the voice said
yes but you must understand
I loved you not despite your great emptiness
but because of your great emptiness—

The Servant

—So you whispered to the soul Rise up!
but the soul was not ready.
—Get up! It's our turn! But that part of the soul
stayed still. So you checked the list

of those who existed

but the soul was not on the list, the soul
responded to none of those things.
Very well, you said. He sank back in his furs.
And you started across the plain to one he loved—

December Shadow

—Then how to address the place where the soul was not.
Should you have said, standing next to the trench,
this should have been you?

This darkness was not the terror of what we do to each other,
or the delicious sexual darkness he'd brought you
or the black corridors of the female body—

remember the early diagrams,
what the inside of a woman looks like?
A cow's skull.

This darkness was the protection of the child,
it included the vast fluttering
as the oak included the moths
with its shadow—

remember in the brilliant day long ago,
the ball coming toward you?
You played with the other children like this—
not *as* anything—
blocked the sun with your non-
being as it were,
but by that pewter shadow you could be affirmed . . .

One by one they kissed you.
One by one the guests advanced themselves
into the night where you would have been
had they looked for you

though it was not in the dim night
that you'd planned to receive them
but at midday, when the druid oak
blossomed with moths, with being gone—

January Dawn

—Two window shades: the stiff
premonition forcing its way around them,
then the first sparrows, chipping through the ice.

And god lies beside you in his—
Wait.   So god lies beside you
in his brokenness
covered with black feathers

and in his claw
a small fish—
shiny and new—like a metaphor.

When Elijah came to the widow of Zarephath
she was by the well—weren't they always
by the well, lowering the gold
rope of consciousness—

Elijah's need in the desert had been represented
by the circle of black ravens
holding fish and they were
dazzling in the text—just dazzling! —and behind them

o the little tents of change O the tents of Ahab's men.

The widow trusted him
though her son died, for Elijah had known
one great moment of faithfulness.

And so
this morning, though you cannot
tolerate your life because it is so
difficult, so   "filled with promise"

think of the spirit of darkness
that did not abandon you,
and the earth that rests outside you, wanting
the form for which it was created—

March Dawn

—Remember the darkness
of the beaten child all your days. Who was meant
to protect her. They hid under the stairs.
The mother clung to her and beat her,
clung to her and beat *her,*
the carefully heard.

So much that child wanted the mother's good opinion
but the mother never spoke well of her,
hating her flesh, its ignorant blood . . .
Motherhood . . . Look: dawn
the color of the pietà. Motherhood
is sorrow . . .

You who do not exist: remember:
darkness created itself
for the child;
she put that poem under the stairs of chaos
but the edge still shines.

See what lies around you; look at his back.
Or at the dusty iris,
the hounds-tongue in the forest.
See your shadow in the dark—still gray grass,
some radiance above it:

everything has a border doesn't it?
the edge where light cannot get in

until joy knows the original wound.

Which is why the earth is feminine,
and the body, not the soul, cries out in heaven—

Blossoms Appearing

—In the pause between
No, wait.
Between winter and the time you greeted it:
plum blossoms. Plum blossoms everywhere!

Always in this season there was this
black self-conscious eye above the landscape,
one feverishly plucked, forties eyebrow
arched like a fermata in music

watching the modern variations in pink
all the way down Euclid Avenue—then

dizzy and with what hope you managed your predicament:
not to lose your shadow to the shared
delirium of each tree.

One day it came to you.
Spring cried as you turned the numb soil.
Earthworms twisted warm cuneiform bodies, arching up
in something—if it was not delight
it was so much like delight—

and a rusty robin landed slowly as an old biplane,

shook the branch, and all
the blossoms fell
on you deliciously it was not sorrow

then you knew for the bird as for you the world
split open was stunningly beautiful
though being alive was nearly impossible—

Every Life

—And right before daybreak the little owl returned:
two small solid o's,
like napkin holders.

Then the briefer, brighter o's of another bird of prey,
not a victim,
came across the field to welcome her.

Dawn has four stages. In the third,
everything chooses how much more it will become;
until then,
the door is the same color as the hinge,

poems fit into other poems, every life
fits into every life,
bright into dark, not deciding.
After that,

the wall notices the shadow pulled out of the soul,
gray as a puritan

and the brave, dreamy hyacinth starts to be seen—

could the garden have said
to the gardener, I made you grow? They were
beside one another.

Could that which was not yet
press forward in the world? It seemed for a brief time
it could—

A Vigil

—Your shadow came to the wall one last time,
        as the lioness comes to the stone gate of heaven.
It was the female ego, fueled by desire.

And you asked: our love, will he always
        be with us? Dawn came in,
weak around the edges, a whorl of parafin.

So you waited, in your creatureliness, crouched
        like an attic rat, you waited till spring,
you loved its glorious imitations

of being alive, young sparrows, their orange scribbles.
        Then you asked again: our love,
will he always be with us?

and the voice behind the voice replied:
        Always. Like yours, his fate was to exist
even against your wall of hope.

So you got up. The islands winked
        red, blue, white, in patriotic
disagreement. Commuters began their orderly

        bright care. Then, E E E,
chiff chiff. Notes from the cypress,
        from one who did not doubt: a jay

sat on top as if he caused the tree to be there—

First Thought

The first thought
was rage—

In certain systems, the point at which that thought
emerges from God's mind is his consort,
but before she turns her rage onto the world, the violent
lords must give her the body of a woman which is not easy.
Imagine them standing around before they will trap
God's vague thought into female flesh. The way
their robes undulate, the slightly yellowing raiment—

poor things.
They will not understand the rage.
It will be expressed forever in the split in things.
In the two-toned lupine,
in the cupped, silk lining of the tulip,
in the red and white of all armies in all wars,
it will bend over my dream wearing his face.

The moment my daughter was lifted
from me, that sticky
flesh screamed fury,
for she, too, blamed the female body—
I loved it that she screamed —

and I knew I had been sent to earth to understand that pain.

The nurses moved about, doing something
over to the left. Probably weighing her
on what looked like blue tin. The flash of non-
existence always at the edge of vision,
and in the next moment, some unasked-for radiance.

Under those lights,
the nurses seemed shabby—
the ivory lords, come haltingly
into the bridal chamber, slightly yellowing raiment.

The last pain on earth will not be the central pain,
it will be the pain of the soul and not the body,
the pain of the body will be long since gone,
absorbed into the earth, which made it beautiful—

don't you love the word raiment?
Dawn comes in white raiment.
Something like that.

II. Dark Matter

*"And immediately Sophia stretched forth her finger
and introduced light into matter, and she
pursued it down to the region of chaos."*

(from "The Hypostasis of the Archons")

Mighty Forms

The earth had wanted us all to itself.
The mountains wanted us back for themselves.
The numbered valleys of serpentine wanted us;
that's why it happened as it did, the split
as if one slow gear turned beneath us . . .
Then the Tuesday shoppers paused in the street
and the tube that held the trout-colored train
and the cords of action from triangular buildings
and the terraced gardens that held camelias
shook and shook, each flower a single thought.

Mothers and children took cover under tables.
I called out to her who was my life.
From under the table—I hid under the table
that held the begonia with the fiery stem,
the stem that had been trying to root, that paused
in its effort—I called to the child who was my life.
And understood, in the endless instant
before she answered, how Pharaoh's army, seeing
the ground break open, seeing the first fringed
horses fall into the gap, made their vows,
that each heart changes, faced with a single awe
and in that moment a promise is written out.

However we remember California later
the earth we loved will know the truth:
that it wanted us back for itself
with our mighty forms and our specific longings,
wanted them to be air and fire but they wouldn't;
the kestrel circled over a pine, which lasted,
the towhee who loved freedom, gathering seed
during the shaking lasted, the painting released
by the wall, the mark and hook we placed
on the wall, and the nail, and the memory
of driving the nail in, these also lasted—

Adult Joy

The slender vessel used for weddings
was also used for funerals.
Loutrophoros. Handles curled
like rams' horns, and beneath some rigid frills,
the ghost-bride greets the master
of the underworld. Are terra-cotta
slaves running around with stylized
gestures on the back of the vase?
Nothing is obvious but that the bride
is confused. What was to be joy
is not continuing. Jagged
lightning designs. Death
greets her like a senator.
I sat last night in a cheap cafe
leaning on the dignity of a small table.
Worn carpet with an eighteenth century
pattern. And all around the room,
bent over silver paperbacks, eating
and being filled, others
like myself, one writing a treatise
on a napkin . . . How
did this sudden joy come in?
Joy by subtraction,
joy in the dim human realm . . .
I thought of Wordsworth's
formal joy fading in fourteen
lines commending him to death
or Herbert's childlike adjunct
to renunciation . . . No, it was
the little adult joy
he'd raised in me, pure, like the tube
of space-time after an accident:
the worst has already happened!
I flattened the book; the plate
of splendid vegetables arrived,
healthy food for the readers

of Berkeley whose faces glow
but not perfectly . . . The owner
slouched behind the counter,
selling his jars of night.
And under a grate on Center,
an iron ladder greeted the revised hell
where the pool shimmered, filled
the space that would transform
the wedding. The death-
bride adjusts her tiara . . . Freud
walks to the desk; his favorite
statue, bronze Athena,
has lost her spear. We grow up.
Joy becomes the missing event,
what reaches us unknown
without wisdom. Joy is the spear.

Food

In a side booth at MacDonald's before your music class
you go up and down in your seat like an arpeggio
under the poster of the talking hamburger:
two white eyes rolling around in the top bun, the thin
patty of beef imitating the tongue of its animal nature.
You eat merrily. I watch the Oakland mommies,
trying to understand what it means to be "single."

*

Across from us, females of all ages surround the birthday girl.
Her pale lace and insufficient being
can't keep them out of her circle.
Stripes of yellow and brown all over the place.
The poor in spirit have started to arrive,
the one with thick midwestern braids twisted like thought
on her head; usually she brings her mother.
This week, no mother. She mouths her words anyway
across the table, space-mama, time-mama,
mama who should be there.

*

Families in line: imagine all this
translated by the cry of time moving through us,
this place a rubble. The gardens new generations
will plant in this spot, and the food will go on
in another order. This thought cheers me immensely.
That we will be there together, you still seven,
bending over the crops pretending to be royalty,
that the huge woman with one blind eye
and dots like eyes all over her dress
will also be there, eating with pleasure
as she eats now, right up to the tissue paper,
peeling it back like bright exotic petals.

*

Last year, on the sun-spilled deck in Marin
we ate grapes with the Russians;

the KGB man fingered them quickly and dutifully,
then, in a sad tone to us
"We must not eat them so fast,
we wait in line so long for these," he said.

*

The sight of food going into a woman's mouth
made Byron sick. Food is a metaphor for existence.
When Mr. Egotistical Sublime, eating the pasta,
poked one finger into his mouth, he made a sound.
For some, the curve of the bell pepper
seems sensual but it can worry you,
the slightly greasy feel of it.

*

The place I went with your father had an apartment to the left,
and in the window, twisted like a huge bowtie,
an old print bedspread. One day, when I looked over,
someone was watching us, a young girl.
The waiter had just brought the first thing:
an orange with an avocado sliced up CCCC
in an oil of forceful herbs. I couldn't eat it.
The girl's face stood for something
and from it, a little mindless daylight was reflected.
The businessmen at the next table
were getting off on each other and the young chardonnay.
Their briefcases leaned against their ankles.
I watched the young girl's face because for an instant
I had seen your face there,
unterrified, unhungry, and a little disdainful.
Then the waiter brought the food,
bands of black seared into it like the memory of a cage.

*

You smile over your burger, chattering brightly.
So often, at our sunny kitchen table,
hearing the mantra of the refrigerator,
I've thought there was nothing I could do but feed you;
and I've always loved the way you eat,
you eat selfishly, humming, bending

the french fries to your will, your brown eyes
spotting everything: the tall boy
who has come in with his mother, repressed rage
in espadrilles, and now carries the tray for her.
Oh this is fun, says the mother,
You stand there with mommy's purse.
And he stands there smiling after her,
holding all the patience in the world.

Holding On

—So, one by one I pull the lice from your red hair.
One by one I try to split them with my fingernails;

no use, they hold on
as they were taught to. Still, they glisten
like heavenly sparks in the morning light
of the bathroom.

I have to pull extra hard on many of them,
use the turquoise, fine-toothed comb
provided by the pharmacy.
They hold on with all their strength:
each has its individual hair to love,
each pus-colored creature
has a genius plan for not leaving you.

I fling the lice out in the air,
thinking how the world despises them,
the other mothers of Berkeley,
and the teachers who have not appreciated their beauty.

And though I've had to poison them again,
I've always understood them,
I also wanted to get that close,
wanted to cling to you in just that manner,
even go back to heaven with you so we won't
have to address this problem of the separate you-and-me,
of outer and inner.

I hope we will have our same bodies there
and the lice will have their same bodies,
that each hopeful tear-shaped egg
will be allowed to cling forever, not be pulled
between love's destiny
and a lesser freedom—

Recycling Center

The labeled bins on the California hillside
catch the glint and quarter-glint of passing cars.
Families pull up with their interesting trash
and start unloading: Here, sweetheart,
this goes over in Newspaper. The bundle
hits with a thud. Diet soda cans
spin almost noiselessly down, and the sun-
permitting bottles from a day's pleasure
are tossed into Mixed Glass by the children
who like to hear the smash, unknowable, chaotic,
as matter greets itself and starts to change.

What mystery is inside a thing! If we peered
into the bin, we could see it waiting there,
could believe everything is alive and specific
and personal, could tell by the tilt of one
bottle against the next that it's difficult
to be singular, to have identity, to keep
an outline safe in the terrors of space.
Even the child knows this. Bye, bottle! she shouts,
tossing it in; and the bottle lies there
in the two o'clock position, temporarily itself,
before being swept into the destiny of mixture . . .

And what if some don't want to. What if some items
in the piles of paper, the orange and blue
envelopes from a magazine sweepstakes, numbers
pressing through the cloudy windows
with our names, some among those pale sheets curled
with moisture, would rather stay as they are.
It's spring; we've thrown away mistakes—
tax forms, recipes, tennis-ball-sized
drafts of poems—that which was blank
shall be made blank again—but what if

that failed letter wants to be a failure,
not go back to pulp, and thought . . .
Or across the parking lot, where light insists
on changing the dull cans, a few cans don't want
to be changed, though they should want to,
shouldn't they, should want to be changed
by light, light which is called sweet reason,
honeyed, spectra, magnitude, light that goes
from the parking lot looking helpless
though it is matter that has been betrayed . . .

All afternoon the bins are carried off
by those who know about where things should go,
who are used to the clatter the cans make,
pouring out; and the families, who believed change
would heal them are pulling away in their vans,
slightly embarrassed by that which refused . . .
The bins fill again with hard substances,
the hills bear down with their fugitive gold,
the pampas grass bending low to protect
what was briefly certain and alive with hope.

The Rat

When I can't write, I go in and play with the rat.
Come on darling.
I open the cage and pick him up under the arms,
loving him so much, though I am his jailer—
the little head strains forward,
the body hangs down till the budlike penis
emerges from the tender belly.
Come on, I say to him,
I'm taking a break;
I'm going to stop trying to find myself in poems.

Probably I'll be having no more children
so when I look in his eyes, which are always clear and wet
like salmon roe
I say my son, all day, my son
and let him do all kinds of things:
put his whole head in my mouth,
eat crumbs in the bed,
shit in the laundry basket . . .

This is the bourgeois view of rats, that they are pleasure;
I have the rats of the poor in my attic—
hard for me to love them—
and the rats of the poor in my dreams,
in the barns of childhood,
eating the hot, closed milky ears of corn
till they are shot over and over,
until their magic skulls light up with flame . . .

Come on darling.
I hold the rat close, too close;
let him dig the pink commas of his claws
into my neck, lie for hours on my inadequate breast—

and then he starts this purring or clicking
such as must occur
at the center of the universe,

the sound acacias make when they split
their seeds on a hot day,
a tiny snap as what is dark and curved
twists into openness—

Sorrow of Matter

The idea that everything is sacrificed to something.
Day after day, this being repeated.
The idea that some things are sacrificed
to vaguer forms
and your job to keep asking where suffering comes from

while you send the children off to school—
between the cries of the hermit thrush
(the 'pay, pay')—
carrying their backpacks full of too much stuff
books imagined to be full of strong color, but now
pulling down to make their backs too straight.

And, never mind,
says one thing in this early migration,
the warbler in the rich person's cypress,
never mind, say the pairs, what we create;

first there was brightness,
then it suffered;
suffering invented shape.

Remember how they taught you to stand
in front of objects? Early on,
in mild cities filled with vanilla, with extra dust,
with curvature; people
had begun to find pulsars at the edge of the universe,
drops of smooth shininess,
—like finding the seeds in an orange—

then they took you to see the huge Christ on the hill,
the god made of broken granite,
and oh how he leaned forward,
you could see it hurt him too,
to be trapped in somethingness, in those tiny mosaics with no blood,
rock eyes without eyelids

and you could offer him only your ability to change
like one of those fast terrified pigeons
that sped to his outstretched arms
and landed, flapping eternally their brief difference,
don't make us, lord, don't make us be like you—

The Spell

—And then a lighter sorrow sheltered me.
For weeks I was under the cloak of an archon
then I saw spring, and the spell was broken.

Today the woodpeckers are nesting near the ridge.
She—the big she—stays all morning
in the lichen laurel, waiting for them to approach her.
She makes her call, "I-am-not-I-am-not"
and the males sound like "whacko-whacko"—

they fly through their own crazy vowels,
they fly saying it.

The other end of the binoculars could be the key.
The world would be smaller, then
the most gleaming changes could go by.

Hops up and down, she wants to
and does, she tries
the mincing footsteps of a geisha. This makes them
speed to her, keeping absent places in their wings:
white spots,
as if the thinking of the apple tree had seeped in.

This world is my twin
but I was not cut from the same cloth, I passed
through the shadow so I could be
amazed at it—

thank you shadow, funny birds,
thank you I don't understand what—

Several Errands

The shoe repairman works behind the married shoes,
his whole hand inside the boot he's shining,
everything cozy in the glass displays, laces paired
on gravel he's spread out in the window, shoes
placed as though they're walking, and beside them
propped up, the wooden tongues of shoe horns, poised
to serve the inanimate world . . . He comes out mildly
attentive, soft accent, possibly a Scottish
childhood, possibly sheep to tend . . . Clear day,
first summer divorced in Berkeley, a time of seamless,
indescribable grief; he waits kindly in his blue apron,
fingering the well-worn inner sole, and I am grateful
for those who serve us knowing nothing of our lives . . .

*

The cleaner waits behind the silver bell;
he's from Cambodia and has free Christian literature
on the counter. He greets me with pleasant chatter,
searches through the coats, some left for years,
he says; they make a soft blue whistle as they circulate
on the ovals like the ones under those automatic boats.
As the clothes pass, little checks and prints under
the whooshing of motion, I see my husband's coat—
how long will I call him my husband—like an old friend
passing by quickly not bothering to greet me. Odd now,
I don't have to pick it up, the serious plaid will go
around between the women's suits and stay all night . . .

*

I watch the young butcher flipping over the young
chicken: he takes one wing and sort of spins it,
first on its back, flinging the trimmed, watery
lemon-colored fat into the trash, then before
he starts on the legs he puts his hand so deeply in
that the finger comes out the neck . . . The other butcher
sets the slab of beef under the saw: the riveting

intricate swirl as the dead flesh pulls away;
he goes off, shouts short words from the deep freeze—
to me or to the carcass hanging by the shank?—
I can wait, but the spaces can't, there's a slight
ticking, then the carcass swings and swings . . .
Somehow I thought we would know everything
through the flesh. Perhaps. But my days have become
spirit. The young butcher splits the chicken
down the back, seems to enjoy the crack of the knife
as it enters the bone, so I try to. Housewives lean
against the cool glass to convey holiday news and he
responds without really looking up; I love that.

*

   oh Berkeley summer mornings, aren't they—
what? past the French Hotel, the glint of tiny spoons
so briefly and soberly allowed to rest on white saucers,
the plums just about over, the agapanthus—"lilies of denial"—
in the center dividers, blooming, or just about to—
like me, hearty and hesitant, not wanting to write it,
not wanting to ruin the perfection of the poem
by writing it . . . At the dentist, the little mirror,
the dinosaur prong is put into the mouth. Mouth:
the first darkness. Nearby: the mobile with straw
eyeless fishes. The dentist will go home to her family,
having briefly reached inside the visible mystery
and found nothing . . . I imagine Wisdom in the text
is like this, creating the cosmos from the mind of God,
looking interested and competent; she touches
the physical place with her prong, and the pain shines . . .

(—a man told me I better think
about my 'system.'
Oh dear! I better
think about my 'system'—!)

Dark Matter

It's good to stand at the head of the tram;
it seems like facing fate. Men and children
stand there mostly, next to the brochure rack
and the older women sit on cushions while
the blond, ski-sunburned guide points out
formations on our left: Red Dog Rock (sandstone
forehead furrowed like a basset hound's)
and KT-22, so mathematical. Below us, mixed
conifers, dazzling hurt granite from which
the basalt flowed, and with us the same confusion
as we rise; joy and terror have the same source.

At the top, families head up the rough trail
to mildly dirty patches of old snow. It's summer;
they want to touch it. Two red-haired boys
throw snowballs at their father. Some women
stand with their hands on their hips,
gazing eastward through infinite space.
Brewer's blackbirds land hysterically among
a mile of newly blossomed mules-ears,
and on a cliff's face, a patch of ice shaped
like a sombrero; today nature seems male.
More forevers and more forevers, and then—

I want to see everything but they say now
most of the universe is hidden;
they call what we can't see dark matter,
those particles straining unprovenly through
what is, sucking gravity from the edge
of galaxies. They're trying to find just one
speck of it . . . Why am I thrilled by the idea
that this hurried thing cannot be caught?
That this huge mountain's filled with it,
billions of it going through me every second.
That as I sit on this log, slightly drunk

from the high altitude, looking at sidalcea
in the sun, in awe of moraines, that
I'm being hit with it. Why love the thought
of being struck by a dark thing clean through.
That the little family throwing snow now
in their innocent ways are being penetrated
by an opposite, the main universe, a huge
allegorical black urgency—and we are nothing
but a rind of consciousness, a mild
excess, a little spare color, and not just us,
the thistles and the asters and the blackbirds . . .

Of course this happened at the start of time,
something had to pull away, and I've been trying
to love the missingness in the middle,
the caves of wounded magic; I've studied
the old terrors every day, the brightness
of the world, have loved the random causes,
have learned the kinds of pain in California,
have known the desire to make from pain
some words that would be beautiful and torn—
and now, I want this wholeness. Here,
the blackbirds swarm upward, and the chipmunk

with one-and-a-half brown stripes takes off
with a prize; the red-haired family hurries
toward the tram under the smooth white ear
of the radar. The mountain seems to push up
through us, asking us to keep its hurt.
Today it seems possible to welcome
wounded matter; the ski-lift chairs,
which have lurched forward, being repaired
all afternoon, guard their incompleteness.
Each black, numbered frame pauses till its turn
then offers its own darkness a ride.

The Hair

—the time when after we make love
he still has one of my little hairs in his mouth.

Propping himself up on an elbow
the hallway light behind him making him look like
a black dandelion
outside an opera house, he uses
his forefinger and thumb
to try to coax the hair from the back of the tongue,

a slight push push
then the little drunken sailor voluntarily but childishly
comes forward . . .

An embarrassing moment even for older lovers.
Two or three attempts at this.
He kisses me once, and in so doing, passes
the hair which was still on his tongue

into my mouth.
This brown shiny S or whatever.
I consider the words it could stand for, then:

sojourner, slim, sagacity;

whatever I have loaned
has been given back to me, the body
inside the soul
he holds, is held by, and is not lonely—

Toll Collector

On the way to therapy or to play across the water
I have to pass the toll collector;
she always has her hand out by the time I get there,
a gray-brown palm with thick lines
which are dull olive-green, like the money.
I seem to get her booth so often that I know her
(in the sense of 'at first sight')
though I've only seen the upper half of the uniformed body.

She faces two kinds of ugliness all day:
ugliness which moves and that which doesn't:
the still white tablets and tubes of the oil company,
thinning this century's black blood,
oil that passes her in one shape or another, either
smooth from the smokestacks
or as amber viscosity, lunging in the trucks.
And behind her back, two kinds of beauty,
beauty that moves and that which doesn't:
the fish-scale surface of the water
and the beaten-egg-yolk yellow of San Quentin.

So much of everything passes her:
valuable campers, trucks of toxins on their way
to the destruction of the earth,
and lovers pass her . . . I've passed her with mine,
chatting, looked across his arm as he hands her the dollar,

but mostly I'm alone in my metal box
holding a hand out to her in hers—

she takes the bill with a slight snap
and when I yell Thanks! (that spattered
exclamation point at the end)
or Hi! (with its expectant i
hooked downward, as if she were supposed to
grab onto the end of it and feel something for me)
she looks at me blankly,

starts unwrinkling the bill at the corners
though the bill isn't too wrinkled,
she only pretends it's wrinkled,
the kind of gesture one might make to kill time
what a friend might do if she wanted you
to stay longer while the water boils
so she could tell you of the new, secret joy
or some special need she has
that you could not possibly meet . . .

In the texts I've read of those who stand guard
at the many entrances of the many worlds
lest the migrating souls go by
with too much weight—it's their job to make sure
the journey goes easily,
the debt assumed by heaven is not too great

and I see sometimes that her face absorbs
whatever trouble is least known to me,
and I am no longer apart from her—
she thinks I have given what I owed,
that now I owe her nothing,
and she has started to gesture
forward to the wet, starry haze of the bridge
where a whole line of cars is disappearing
as I must disappear, and the one after me—

III. Gnostic Heaven

". . . at the sound of his voice I awoke and arose
from my slumber and directed my steps that I
might come to the light of our home—"

(from *The Hymn of the Pearl*)

"Do you hear voices?"
"Yes."
"What do they say?"
"The other side of what I'm thinking."

(in a Berkeley clinic)

Gnostic Heaven

Impossible to know much, but it seems they thought
heaven was thick. One illustration
shows the cosmos as a kind of metal onion;
heaven is the outer half. A wedge-shaped
section has been lifted out so we can imagine them
traveling sideways and paradise starting
before they know it, before the smoky orbits
of the planets, before the speckled, fixed stars
and the achromatic rope of the leviathan,
that they've already arrived
at the outskirts of the kingdom of light.

It's Friday afternoon, and in bad traffic
little headaches have started among the drivers.
So much of their shapeless need shows then.
Busy with their radios, they hardly notice
right before the bridge the exquisite
slag heaps rise and glitter. These hills
change only slightly from week to week
or change in relation to each other,
like siblings; some shimmer more,
some less, or a particular glint
will be transferred from an eyeless fender
to a sheet of aluminum that frees and cancels
the light with no help from the sun.

All day bright cranes have worked this scene
and not been noticed. One has a flag
on its elbow. The orange, lace-necked one
has a shovel a child could feel at home in.
The sensitively-strung, pinkish lift
with the platformed man at the controls—
oh—so high!—has caliper hands that sense,
in the simple scraps of cars and ships,
what each was meant for, the intransigence
of certain objects, the refusal

of many earthly forms . . . And the workers in boxes
of scratched glass are like the archons
inventing matter, trying to decide what goes where,
should they make categories, or just
be engaged by the steady rhythms of lyrical arms.

And the travelers, stalled in traffic, are talking
about their days, letting the different weights
of information fall as those on the site
grow casual about their mortal work,
not governed by intent or reason . . .
It's six o'clock. Behind the man's face
something glistens from a hook. Behind
the woman's face, all that mild distance.
They talk and talk. They go over
each bent damaged detail of the week,
and in the accreting power of conversation,
as the slag is gently lifted by the magnet,
the broken days begin to seem whole . . .

So when the entrance shines without warning
it's easy to see why they didn't notice
fixed as they were on each other's eyes—
they didn't realize it would start
before the tollkeepers and the watchhouses
and the storms of knowledge, that the used world
would usher them in with the patience
of metal, the prongs in the dirt all red
and silver, the claw held almost daintily
to show that the brutal, falling thing
was beautiful and welcoming, it was.

*"How can I be distinguished from her? Only if I keep on pressing
through to the other side, if I'm always beyond, because on
this side of the screen of their projections, I can't live . . ."*—Luce Irigaray

Magdalene

"I dreamed god shone—No,
that's not right. I dreamed God
shone his light
upon us and he was jealous. No:

I dreamed God shone the light of his violent miserable longing
upon us and he was
pleased. For once. But the light
was not.

It was the light that used to come from certain houses
east of here. And God, the pinpoint
into which the light
retracted, held it steady, taking our happiness

back to the secret blackness of his Fame . . .

After that, how could I
believe in freedom? When a group
of sparrows rises from the dust, the whole flock shudders
but one stays,

and that is the only one
that interests us: loneliness
through which the truth passes
to complete itself."

      . . . only half believing in it.
      Or half-believing in the female voice,
      so that's one-quarter belief in a way, enough to revive
      the dead forms of religion and love . . .

"There appeared unto me this morning a little goat
with angel wings—jagged, sawtoothed wings, you know the kind,
and its face was smashed in . . .
king

solitude,
bright axis,
I have not been like the others—
(No that's not right, I have been)

king solitude, when they walk by your side
their faces bright with hope,
and you send them back to the miracle of their bodies,
they don't want those tired miracles:

the problem of the swine
or the issue of blood;
they want their permanent hungers,
they want you . . .

Look here.
It will be written down.
You do not have to write it."

     It should have been quite easy to find her.
     I searched a long time.
     It should have been quite easy. To find her
     in the middle of the night while the rose bush struck
                     the window with knotted blossoms,

     and the moon carried the orange coffin of its former light,
     and the free newspaper was hurled from the street:
     whack:
     like that.

     So few women in the text.
     I used to run my fingers over the maps in back,
     the lands of bondage and wanderings,
     those sickly pastels,

being careful not to tear the pages
or she would have to bring the scotch tape,
the yellow kind because it was the fifties,
the kind that cracked like memory and would not
                                    yield with time . . .

Here it is.
The alabaster box.
The Hair.
And they murmured against her.

"I dreamed we were sitting in the garden
and you were pleasing everyone;
your thick wrists made an X over your knee
and I wanted to wash you with my hair . . .

there are those who need everything
and those who can't be served; that's
what we are. We're both whores."

    Think of them sitting in the garden like that.
    Now,
    take him out.
    There. Just leaving her. She has

    a bit part shattered by devils.
    And the place he was—his shape was where
    perfection might have started, if perfection were.
    The man is one. The woman is zero. Or two . . .

"So how does it feel when the power leaves your body?
When you give yourself away?
You think you can help them by listening
and you *can* help them sometimes until you become them,

then the crazy ones start yelling because not
being in their skin hurts them, or having you in there
hurts them—stand up a minute. Let me be you just one second.
I know you are very busy."

. . . and the woman doesn't believe in words;
she pulls a thread at the end of the poem
and mutters to herself as it comes undone.

"I dreamed I saw God dead. No,
come on. I dreamed God's burned body
lay in the desert
and you covered him. But he went on
dying in his obsessive way;
sometimes he raised his head and told anecdotes.
Sometimes he just lay there
hurt and playing God—"

The way everyone is stiff if they haven't been
                        to a parade.
Awkward: the not-
knowingness of them. Only a few were told.
The slapping of the palm fronds as he entered town.

I used to imagine him dragging his feet on the ground.
The donkey was too low.
The manger donkey next to the shepherds.
Then the sickening thought of all those clothes
                        in the dirt . . .

"—and maybe you were waking in that bare little room;
it was time for you to go. A triangle
of light was held by the low
resentful force I called God;
some athletic angels climbed over the ledge
and signaled you to come too: what right
did you have to be inside, they asked; what
was the world's blunt radiance without you?"

Meridian Plinth

The gravestone-looking slab donated to the college
for instructing students about light and dark
and the rotation of the world stands solemnly
in the courtyard being landed on by buff-colored
sparrows with shining breasts and claws. It is
summer in the suburbs and the voices of students
seem to travel a long way from the field
as light has had to travel from far off
to abide in this rock. Two steel pegs
and a chart that looks like a quarter of a pie
etched into the granite will show the passage
of the sun, and in the grooved triple name
of the donor, in the E for east and W for west,
in the other grooves flecked by mica today
the light from noon looks a bit forlorn.

The seven-souled vestments of the flesh
were supposed to keep light in mankind. Secret
names should have been learned by now to ease
its passage home, but were not learned.
And the sun striking down at noon like this—
because it insists on moving—the sun
seems ancillary to the stone, and weaker;
it has to move and last forever, or a little less
long than the imagination. If you stand
very near the plinth you can feel the stored
heat of its mass, and the different kind of light
being saved for you. The parallel worlds
are stacked up and rub against each other,
the worlds we read of in the texts that have to fit
neatly inside each other, one after another,
like a child's bathtub blocks fit, or as your
lover fits. It is the same in the universe:
surely the dark world holds the other close;

and when the time comes, something from outside fate
will come to retrieve the divine sparks.
As dandelions travel from the dry hills today,
or the woman with the baby, coming across the lawn:
maybe *they* are the redeemers. Remember
how the heavenly messengers sometimes
look like tourists, arriving unawares, and after
they feast they become special. When all
the sparks have been retrieved, the cosmos
will be finished, the milky light of the suburbs
cleared of blossoms, of physical terror,
and of doves with their responsible
white shears, trimming the fabric of the day . . .

But of the suffering inherent in matter,
what shall we say? That it goes back
when we go back? That it will die when we do?
If it goes there with us how far away?
Perhaps it will be left, and the plinth
can hold it for us, and go on with its job
of being patient in the sun while the mountain
makes more irreducible granite, more of itself.
The plinth was meant to please and instruct,
holding odd shards of radiance inside;
it wants to live. Stand next to it.
In the other noon, it casts no shadow.

Autumn Moon

. . . the moon comes up in her
secondness, left edge not
filled in quite, the abject not filled in quite
    but trying . . .

•

The infinitely 'being called' then
not chosen,
also the fear of being surpassed, cast
off, you know, not needed . . .

•

When first he—no. When you
first stepped from the restaurant, your
    bodies annointed with peppermint and sweet
herbs, a sliver of moon snagged on his lip . . .

•

She said
it helps to know
Van Gogh with his
obsession for yellow—

•

He tried the windows and he tried—
nope.
    He tried the windows *then*
    he tried the doors.

•

haiku in translation it would be like this

autumn moon colon
some wine stains on white linen
his separate past

•

. . . and the sense
of those dear, fugitive hours, all
erased, erasable!
Still . . .

•

Through the tic-tac-toe of the steel
window grid, the start
of one gold O
then the game is given up—

•

Some heavy, hopeful
woolen clouds over it—
no use.
The Democratic party . . .

•

—and kept working hard on this
instead of the one about
the father, who was, of course,
'the sun'

•

—and saw some swirling
mist over it, notes from
ex-wives over the years, their gracious
almost stupid handwriting—

•

female creativity, avoiding
    the issue of talking
    about the father who was
of course 'the sun'

•

Halloween: with your tiny one
you stand on the curbside,
beam the flashlight up to its
tin cathedrals—

•

the desire to be
        understood though being
        understood was not
what you meant . . .

•

Raindrops off the eaves
make the cage
for the waning moon,
the satisfied one . . .

•

A rich word
used casually in conversation
('inveigled') swells
as you use it through the days

•

When it really is very
crescent, *Die
Valkerie,* the memory
of large, bruised women—

•

calcium
butterin
halcyon
aspirin

•

Sometimes over Tomales Bay at its half
the blue has leaked in through the lace
edge so it really looks unfinished
like a feminine—what?—something

•

—so why *every*
month the white expansion,

that tyrant
    drop of estrogen?

•

    . . . and how could you not have reflected him?
When you were called into the lubianka of the soul,
the question chamber you yourself contained,
it was always he who was there . . .

•

    Passing Kehoe Beach
spotted moon with moth-
        spotted hawk
under her

•

    then in your dark
corner of heaven, to learn
the beauty of your life,
you had to leave something out . . .

•

Woman poet—hateful term!
Sometimes you despised
the moon with her
hymn of granite—

•

three quarters gone
in the faded sky: his Levi's
button
just unbuttoned

•

Send it back!
Send back what was on the right,
the shadow of the feminine, the pastel.
She wasn't nice now, was she.

•

—order within an incompleteness, the cut
tip of a scallion.
Women poets don't have world views,
said the male poet—

•

hard isn't it. Almost full again.
If you press gently
at the edges, at
the dark spots in the poem, it may

spring open—

(—then I asked how
far should I go.
Go deeper, the voice said;
it was double—)

Steinberg Case

hiding girl

. . . the sounds
of morning, of people
succceeding, of people helping
others to succeed . . .

you crouched in the closet, you were
    a good little girl, you had done
one of everything;

it will become
clear to you why you
offered yourself to your own destruction

believing he was all
    power and consequence—or didn't
offer, no, that's not it, go on now—

Isaac put himself on a slab
thinking he owed him something
in an eternity based on sacrifice;

    and doesn't fear give the child
some position in space?
                  because at the edge
of your becoming, something kept trying
to erase you . . .

        the implicate
   gold, the violin-
      brown of your hair . . .

the closet

. . . so you could not be
punished for not having tried;
that was the main thing . . .

       and in the closet, with your
'bad attitude'
       you could make yourself fit anywhere:

into the crevice where winter begins
       or the Y where the cypress
unbraids itself

or the plane where the shadow sees
just how to live: it hovers
       underneath the sulphur butterfly.

The truth of the wound
is a narrow truth . . .
you could go like the worm

back to the pre-earth, stay there for years
       fitting neatly against the sides,

come out with a double hope: first to enter
the room as a girl, let's say,

—then, not to be recognized!

elusive one

. . . and the poem wanted
to be just like you! it agreed
to erase itself . . .

                He stood quite near
in the quaint, positive rooms
looking down at you as someone looks
at a stain on a new shirt, perhaps,

not hoping to get it out
but hoping someone *else* will get it out . . .

It will become clear
to you why you
offered yourself to your own destruction

believing he was all power and consequence

though he made his hands
      into fists his hands
meant to hurt you he
didn't didn't didn't didn't mean to did he—

and you looked up at him
      with all your childish logic,

you who did not rank among the saved . . .

killed shadow

. . . don't avert
your eyes from what
you cannot bear:
                    that the child gathered
herself up in her joy, was playing,

then she—
no. Then he dug a trench
in her body and put his childhood into her.

And now, peer into her. Isn't it
        your face there, in the wide look
of the dead girl,

in all the world that wears his darkness: old
        speeding cadillac on the bridge, twin
        darknesses fitting under
the lip of the fender, in the drugged
redhead's ripped
fishnet stockings on Telegraph: poor beaten wretch.

—From the split
yawn of the cypress, summon the cry.
Summon the memory into which
        you cannot vanish further,

you who endured
the terrors of your life
in his name . . .
                    all right then. That's
fine then. What you can't
recall   shall be your instrument . . .

extra life

I will cry out as the strap
to him and to all time
I will not go

I'd rather be manifest as air
than hurt a child . . .

So many years later.
She is gone and it's
possible to be of two minds about this,

too often inspecting the place of the wound . . .

I wanted to forgive him, that's not the problem.
But pain like a vector passed into the earth;
too fast the living move over it.

Generation upon generation of this
and someone will have a childhood;

but still in the dark
I hold the abject one, who says
I will come out now because the day invites me:

the ellipsis of the carpenter's nails,
three black taps,
the stars of milk in the coffee . . .

Small Spaces

—And the earth was still baffled by the small spaces,
especially in spring
when people admired its growth from great heights.
The earth was baffled by the tiny gaps
suchs as those between minutes.

In those places of yearning,
as in the emptiness between
a child's back teeth, it was trying to decide
if there should be any later.

If so how much later.

Not even wild cypresses by the bay
move firmly enough to satisfy the small spaces.
The moon swells, and does its part. Purple vetch
and smart lupine
combine to think it through, too many
get ready and a few die daily to fill the spaces—
stem after short stem—

though the earth tried to hold each one of them upright,
saying don't imagine don't imagine
there has been another like you—

for my mother

untitled fragments

(—Who wounded you, my love.
Who took your secret shadow. Who brought you
to this place   dear night plus day.

And now, nothing sleeps as you sleep
bruised spark, since you've become matter,
since you've fallen to the wide earth, to
                              sleep near me . . .

You whom I call you:
whatever touched you, whatever got in the way
I loved that too,

the kiss of the other person, the little extra
redness on the throat of the finch,
my horizontalness, your verticality—)

(—How long will you stay here.
Maybe longer. Sometimes,
the bee has so much pollen, it can't fly!

and lands on the drunk camelia.
I watched you sleep,
delicious flesh, I watched you rise,

you made the dawn jealous,
you kept the future of the day inside,
not showing,—

And when you left, you were
so everywhere!   torn spark. The night
had used you up, but you kept going—)

(—Why did you tremble when you came in here.
I saw some doves fly the city;
this place, had no door.

You came in with your old sorrow,
with your other sexual loves in your mouth
your wrong previous your two laters

their little silver crosses in your eyes,
I wanted to be the boy,
I would have loved you against the wall
                as hard as I could,

but there was no I right then,
desire is the good general,
the wall was nearly gone—)

(—While I slept you stood
in the colorful night market
with pyramids of bright fruit piled high

where those who loved you
rushing back to their intimate stalls
held out the pears that had been dreamed for you.

And, would the dream pear not come gladly
once it knew this was you
wanting to take it in?

The dream pear chose reality
wanting your mouth, as I did—honestly,
it was happy to be bitten—)

(—In the cave of the self
the light shines only so far. After that
you have to crawl.

I searched for you and everything you touched
was magic half in bloom twice not knowing
whether to begin at the center or not.

Why look for happiness outside yourself.
Because, that's why. The entrance
to the cave was still far off.

We traveled 'by night' and slept 'by day'
perpendiculars rushing past and we were two
animals with western eyes waiting to cross
                          the highway—)

A Foghorn

On Sundays in mid-winter, when wild iris
put their iridescent blades through the grasses
and yellow lupine wait to flower from their seven-
fingered hands, all the divorced Californians
start out to the Point with their bottled waters
in their fragile foreign cars; they pass the turn-off
for the hopeful murmur of beaches, and pass
the moody grays of cooperative farms, the cattle
with their useful udders the color of wild geranium;
then they park if they can and descend the long steps
by the lighthouse where the tough crimson algae
cling to the broken stones, and when they arrive
at the rail they look past the cormorants, past
the Farallones to the space where the whales should be,
and the split chord of the foghorn calls to them.

The whales are too far to hear it; the whales,
in their secrecy, give off the dull sheen
of Etruscan mirrors. Down the coast they travel,
and the twisted cypresses gather to look: they swim
by L.A., with its nights of shining leather, toward
the temperate waters of Baja where they will mate.
In pictures, they are all smiles: sweet diligence,
or the weak little smile of exhausted history.
Their corrugated sides undulate as they play,
moving in a time both linear and cyclical.
They all swim here: Melville's whale, and Jonah's—
even the hollow plaster whale of Disney—
for this is California. Surely the people crave
some blankness between sightings, but someone
spots one every few minutes: a heart-breaking flash,
the cry goes out—each moment a contained unit—
then the cry passes, brief as a human life.

They say the call is heard in all the great systems.
The sleepy ones have gathered at the shore

to proclaim the glamour of the alien sun,
while in the nearby desert one real solitary
arranges himself on a pile of fronds . . . Come home,
says the disembodied voice to all of them.
But here on the Point the wind is fierce;
it blows the people to the right as they pose
for snapshots under the beehive-shaped, art deco
lantern, and the foghorn calls their two-toned names
until the names sound interchangeable: John-ny! Mar-y!
a major third downward, accent on the second syllable.
The call goes out in reverse, away from them,
over the hugely populated universe as though
it sent their questions out for them:
What shall we be? What shall we do now,
divorced from our lives, and from this century?

And the land splits behind them, the conglomerate cliffs
letting them go, letting the Point slide toward Alaska.
They wait as if at the prow of a fatherless ship,
leaning there; they have waited a long time,
they are so used to waiting, they have waited for
the winning number, or for the changes in someone,
or for the nocturne to rewind itself around the spool—
shouldn't something have pity on them now?
It is late; pelicans and egrets and herons go by,
and the foghorn continues its anthem of names, only
for them, of course, only in this human realm.

IV. Bright Existence

"If there were no unevenness, then we would have
only one nature. But, as unevenness exists,
they have made you a man, and me a woman."

(from a Gnostic Mandaean text)

"The shadow can be realized only in relation to a partner."

(C. G. Jung)

"There are mysteries hidden still in the bedrock of
Point Reyes; origin and age are two of them."

(Jules Evens, *The Natural History of the Point Reyes Peninsula*)

Trapped Light

I knocked at the door of my life
and someone was already there,
standing in a future I had not thought to build,
speaking words I hoped to recognize.

For years I woke beside him
in the dark, studied
the tiny hairs on his back. Some
left, some right, like sea babies. They moved
around in their direction.

Light came over the window ledge, passing itself by. What
could it do, loving only
its opposite. Got stuck in the bent-over
dust motes, the little furnace. Got stuck
in the hairs on his back.
What could I do with the old need for entrapment.
The tragedy (and gift) of not
being the other person. The gift of not being
in the same body 'as he.'

I lay in the bed or the room of my life
where my brief shadow had not slept
and watched the night come down and touch his eyes

till waking, I was called out of myself

and in place of the old blindness
were the eyes of a new face tired with wonder
and in place of the soul's deaf question, was a voice—

Vast Fluttering

I walked with my traveler through a long system of valleys
at the end of summer
under a non-moon. Crowns
of periwinkle. Mint. Dusty laurel. The scent
of the nearly finished, about to become—

And those tiny loud berries were hardest at the end of summer
coming forward to be finished
—not having enough existence to be ripe
(yet full of crimson crimson hope)—
the white blossoms that would not fruit
were powdery at the center,
moon-powdery like the sixties, and the blossoms
came forward as trapped light.

What is the uncertain part that wants to be finished by another
What little uncertain part comes forth in thorns
each thorn hooking back to not
being a cardinal's crest
What uncertain part comes forth in thorns

(Some moths with old-lady-curtain-wings flew by)

And I loved my traveler but I feared his bright edges
the manner in which he
, looked off to the side. At mother nature.
Loved my traveler quite a lot
though he carried the past on his back—her blond changes—
and seemed at ease while I was keeping watch,
(split and puzzled and keeping watch)
he seemed at home in this bright accident,
so what was my almost compared to his being there,
my half-darkness compared to his complete light,
my local compared to his everywhere
and what was I   Was I.   (Was I)

The notion of fate pulling us sideways
Fate which traps light in the alders
Causes the vast fluttering of the supposed-to-be-there
Fate which turns young ladies into trees
and put the plague of the oak moths up that year
I loved him so outside myself I didn't fear, for several minutes!

(moths with ragged curtain wings flew by)

And the little identity owl said Fool, Fool
The archbishop of couldn't said Why, Why,
Some little nightingale-type-thing said
How previous of you

—moths with mended curtain wings flew by.

I had some boxes of noon I carried around inside
a little lit room sealed up by several dawns
I'd been reading some books on female identity
but who was I (Was I)
Had received the gifts of the new privacy
like women of my decade
Had absorbed the freckled glow of the moon in detail
But what was my little lit room
Compared to his little lit room
My sometime compared to his every single time
What were my shelves on female identity
And what was I (was I)

The problem of falling in love in this century.
The problem of it not being
natural anymore. No no not that they said no more
popular yearning. You must be in relation
to him something finished.
But I saw nature looked completely unfinished
Ellipsis and :   :   :   of the cicadas
Half of an owl (maybe only one wing). Mostly
things had been omitted.

Mostly I heard mostly mostly
in the Katharine Hepburn pines.

What is the part that wants to be matched by another
What part wants to be seen clear through
Doesn't want nature as the mother exactly
or wants the dark rising
colorless cobra female, the end
We walked through night till night was the poem
Night after night I felt three necessary valleys between his knuckles
Night after night, his hand stayed in my hand

An osprey stood by its possible nest.
It looked like an ace of spades standing there
sleeping. Backlit. Its neck in its pocket.
Sprigs of slightly shabby sticks it had arranged
after a casual tour of oceans.
And we loved that dark bird together,
it brooded, looking the very dawn at us,
its grief cry tucked in, for later use,
now only the gutteral R of high school French
to put itself to sleep

but so much pure creation packed around its lucky nest,
a slight, then a vast, vast fluttering;

and we loved that dark bird, together we were the bird,
he loved the center of what had already happened
and I loved what it was becoming—

so the future stretched before us as a series
of perceptions

and I saw how loving a thing beside him
I might become extra
not so less, not so unnumbered,
that loving a thing beside him I might become two—

Almost Shadow

If immortal love exists,
why then this terror. The terror
of the other, being too near . . .

And not only that: of even
walking beside the other person.
You'd ask around. Maybe you weren't
the only one to feel this.

Summers especially, when dawn is loud,
when you hear at their fullest being,
proud, elegant juncos fighting over the millet,
the jays, the teenage sparrows
who can't stay on the branch with one another,
then flutter (almost) to the ground
in love with having fallen;

such had been the case for you.
Finding yourself loved or loving, you felt the fear
(as though a frontier
lantern had been held up)
        of being almost too dim.

That being an almost
was the same as being
nothing. You know, being
nothing, in relation to him—

Spare World

I walked with my traveler through several infinities
beside the estero
under the gray sun. Always the fox
sparrows lifting autumn through their bodies. Crows
in their judge robes flew overhead

and the dirt shone
our laughs were tied together,

the milky white birdshit with the purple tinge of
—(they had been eating berries)—heaped up
around the owls' clover.

And I loved my traveler but I feared his completeness,
the way everything kept
, taking him in. And everything took me in
because I was beside him. One ragged
cypress leaning sideways, as it did.
Even the lightning struck, the previously glorious.
Even the stumps of the oak were receiving of us, then.

—Old Mr. Black-beetle crossing the trail
where is your mate you shiny thing

But for my part I noticed everything was split
(because of the divorce or the fault line probably)
Even two colors of gray in the granite.
Each set of needles in the bishop pine
short deliberate pairs
thrust from the papery wrappings at the end,
no pair wanting to be just one needle,
both halves wanting to be separate;

and the hemlock at this time in summer
has this separate, sort of dry interior,
like styrofoam.
Makes it rattle, almost.

But, there is no way to tell you how beautiful he was,
climbing the dry hill,
holding the unplanned bouquet of the several dying grasses
which had come to him,, of course, so willingly—
wild wheat wild rye wild barley
Each with its split dialectical seed
(split but not divorced, split but orderly)
he held with his sexual hand those agreeable grasses
—seeds falling off them,

the ambassador of outside, the source of gladness—

and the meadows hurried brown,
the greatly unstressed fields turned middle-aged and handsome,
not wanting to be themselves anymore;
the grasses wanted to be just like him.

O.K. but.
How to walk beside another person,
was what was wrong with me.

(Or, not wrong exactly.
Just like the women of my era.)

Birds of the estero could walk beside.
Greater yellowlegs stepped goldenly
beside the willet.
Could could (could) Could. Goldenly
toward the one gleaming trout.
Surely the willet could manage on its own,
two dark wing smudges holding it up
(could, could, could) The briefly
seen. My love stood beside;
I watched him plain who watched a flock of
(according to him) sandpipers

turn together 4 ways, like a box
—gray white black nothing—
they turned together 4 ways
like a box mailed out to sea

79

and as he took my hand
I felt the split in nature mend
not because I learned, the split learned;
I tried to cross to count his otherness
and when I couldn't count
it counted,
that bright love counted me—

(—Faster messed up poor only
helper go
faster, and the soul said sorry
my this one I can't go any faster—)

Branch, Scraping

—In the almost city of new joy you lay awake.

Open up dark me, you said (having waited),
part that lives on the inside of statues
holding those poses
half-covered with reverse dust,
part that barely lives,
open up open up open up, you said,

(because you knew how much activity lives in the night,
the rats, thrumming
and thrumming their violin ways up the sides of dawn,
new roses climbing
up the edge of fiddle this and fiddle that)

And the dark me said
I can't come right now let me put on further shadows
I am a torn thing—

The dark boys were wakeful so you asked them
The sad boy the mad boy the see-you-later
sailors sailing backward
track marks under their tans
husbands of people brothers of people the wild boy
the spinning man
the dream pirate who loved night so well
he had to stir tomorrow in his coffee . . .

There was a branch scraping so you blamed it,
its thorns advanced by little yellow roses.
Civilization was scraping so you blamed it
(tearing the female from himself and the male from herself;
there was a branch scraping between worlds so you blamed it

and the day people slept on their thoughts,
the branch scraped midnight
because the noon ones slept.

So o.k., maybe it. Maybe nature
wasn't always such a good mom. Maybe she was sick
of doing whites in her laundry. Maybe
she was a he—

(Try this sentence backward
: he a was she maybe) Dirty boy-boy.
Raccoons searched through the garbage can,
pulling out chicken bones, live sandwiches,
the little bloody pad
of black black purple-black black female blood
—What did he want that for,
his eyes were ringed with it—
and the owl did its four note call
from ahead of the wrinkled moon:
(dirty) who-who . . (dirty) who-who . . .

Branch scraping.
Branch scraping again. It made the sound
of missingness, like you. It made
the sound of tiny eiffel towers on their sides.
But was it the dark girl
or the dark boy self you were missing.
Doesn't matter what it was about. Dirty moon-moon. Little
drugged missionary stars came out.

So you took their advice and stayed awake in half
as in a tunnel where you are the only one
going the opposite way,
—not so yellow, not so open,—
you come out and the trees have split
between the past with its type of fire
and the future with its,
you can burn through one sweet branch at a time,
you can gather up the branches with your large large heart
but you're not going to be one thing, ever again—

Archaic Wanderings

I walked with my traveler
and thought of the other women before me.
Probably they'd looked at those very same grasses together,
hairgrass, foxtail, barley, who
cares, so what if they had;
willows dropped their blonde eyebrows.

In childhood, I had this map called Canaan
at the Time of Conquest.
That was before I knew the Kennedys did it,
before any sex at all.

Minuscule names of tribes slanting
into each other,
the mouth-wrinkles smiling around the Dead Sea;

the thought of all those boys and women
with cloth and the long hair and the many directions,
striped tents,
the vast fluttering, the whisper
of airy things being lifted off, the warm
dry mouths of strangers being kissed;

sex stays fairly secret
for a long time, doesn't it. That map
had pale yellow skin,—like many of my wrists—

Torn Shadow

—In the minor city of black joy you lay awake.
And, you could just about
go out there, couldn't you,
torn shadow.
Part that was almost loved.

But who would have noticed you.
Would the wind with its nada nada,
or the moon with her acne scars, would she,
or the tulips, whispering too loudly
for you to join them
or the mommy darkness? Not really.

You went out to the night city,
you went suffering again. You called
to the night city, you called suffering again,
and midnight came with its twelve dancing princess type of thing,
the dark boys brought their shadows past the bed,
: the daddy the brother the drug-boy
the hunger the meaning
junkie who read magazines standing up for free
the nice scholar the not-nice scholar
the wild boy of suppose
poet one poet two poet B
and the dream pirate who loved night so well
he wore his bracelets like the moon
and stirred the afternoon into his tea, and

you asked them why
wasn't I loved and the dark boys said, nyeh nyeh
you didn't want to be.

But the dark boys loved the won't part, didn't they.
You know the won't part:
won't work won't shit won't love
serene gifts round beaches the so-called

light of day. Most of the universe is filled with it,
it seems like. Dark matter, lamb fat,
Tuesday night television.
The won't part won't go away.

(So you asked again why wasn't I loved,
and the dark boys said
we had a torn shadow, how could we have been.)

Nights at the marina, thick with fishermen there,
their buckets full of pliant perch,
you can fly over the city,
see the rejected shadow, the him and the not-him.
Marlboro smoke makes pewter fences between the men,
beer bottles with paper bags bunched down
around the mouth-places,
and the shadows lie faithfully flat beside their owners
in the medium neither;
what could be darker than the male shadow at night
before it is plucked up by gulls, (, all
both of them) and dropped into the famous sea—

(So you asked again
how can I love if I was not loved
and they said, you can lie down in your emptiness now
if you want to.)

At night the prison glows like the back of the Mona Lisa.
The men make sexual deals with each other.
The beautiful swagger,, (as if that's bad)
the locomotive tattooed
on the back of another (as if that's bad)
the man bends over the sink spitting,
the hurt and the extra senses clouding his blood,
they want to televise his execution,
televise his face as he slumps down,
they show the picture of the man he killed,
he says he would do it again, over and over . . .

Torn shadow,
dark boy,
doomed male energy,

you spoke well when you were young,
you blended in with the night
when they told you to; you acted strong,
so why didn't they. Why
didn't they love you.

Marshy Area

I walked with my traveler and thought about time,
thought of it arriving
over the rim of consciousness,
that the farthest galaxies get younger
as they speed off from us
in lights the color of sixties lipgloss,
that consciousness has only one voice
which continues utterly
and I wanted it forever for my own . . .

Standing by in the marshes: eternity and a few phoebes,
the nests of woodrats piled high with sticks,
thick medicinal cattails,
and blackbirds rose in polyvalent song,
a song just about the strength of fishing nets;

and I wanted to go on walking
away from cities like this,
casting off raffle tickets and approximations
where the needy kept pulling us,
without time with him as my freedom,
though I was too close to be loved,
I wanted to see, not apart from this other being
the smart and actual motions of the clouds—

Useful Shadow

—In the practical city of plaid joy you lay awake.
How could you listen
to all of them, anyway. Why was it you
you couldn't love.

You lay on your right side
with your twelve darknesses, you lay on the left
with your historical calm;
earthworms tied the middle corners
of the garden. The moon
lay on her back with her sharp enthusiasms.

So,,. What kept you awake. Must have been
the sense that you had to do something useful. That you had
to perform to get love.
Revised lists were being sent
at this very minute, matter of fact. Lists
of important things you hadn't done,
because weren't you the boss's little helper?
For him you carried the olive branch,
cast the golden calf, invented
farming, invaded small countries, wrote checks
to the Contras, Oliver
North in his bullet-proof vest
plus all the members of Congress saying, You really
don't remember, Mr. North?
(the useful shadow draped over his chair
so it could be worn at press conferences,
wash 'n' wear shadow)

—you think you have no Oliver in you?
you were daddy's little helper,
you tried so hard like reality, and now
you wondered what they'd use you for.

Boy prostitutes must think like this.
Coastal pine trees must wonder
why being good tall pine trees isn't good enough,
why they have to be used
for something else, a coffin or a table or paper to wipe shit on.

Handsome nothing
standing at the heart of matter
with your self-hate and your twelve month contract:
no one was checking. Before
you'd done a single thing, you were enough.—

Luminous Textures

I walked with my traveler in the silver conditions
toward the middle of winter
beside the lagoon. Pods of finished
lupine, approving, rattling nicely. I had never
—let's see. I had not been
so this outside with anyone—

—he had such good posture, like a meadowlark,

and the meadowlarks themselves (the hero-looking
black footprints on their chests
clicked their tails shut shut open shut.

How do you learn to love another person.
Was this my possibly. Might have been,
but still. I mourned
the idea that I was not him,
wrapped in the long changes,, a sympathizer,

and feared the earth loved him
better than me (because he was so
far outside   (I feared
the earth loved him better than me.

Not so whispered the missingness.
Not at all rattled the dried.
But it takes such work to open the heart even a little,
pretty much most of a life.
Look at this will you. So many shadows
on the outside—black stripes on the goldfinches,
warblers with their lone ranger masks on,

and so many shadows in the pre-lagoon area,
grasses shone into which they flew,
spikelets, panicles and the long awns
reaching into the sometimes,

I envy texture,
that it can be right and wrong at the same time,
outer and inner, that it can be "next to"—

what if I just did that, a little.
What if I just stood close to him, like texture.

It's more the men
who like to stand gazing at the waterfowl
—(buffleheads and one big smart ruddy duck).
It's more the women who understand the lagoon.
Says to itself,
watch me hold more. Says to itself,
(, ,) all night I needed boundaries, love.
I was scared of being the ocean.

And the shine kept pulling off the luminous textures:
outside inside out I'm all confused.
Come on in said the willing underground.
Open up, just a little.

There are those in whom creation seems extra;
he was one of those.
Hard not to get lost in him like a dime on the beach
if you kept feeling bright
as you sank down—
(now the dime is a you.
The problem of falling in love is: the pronouns go.

On the beach, bumpy starfish were clinging to each other.
Kelp tangled up in itself like doomed languages.
Whales sounded and surfaced, heading toward Magdalena,—

but you had been threatened by doubleness and extra,
were soothed by singularity,
had wanted to be strong in the middle, like a Wednesday,

maybe you could just.
For five minutes. What if you stood
beside him just a little.

All right went the agencies of eagerness,
dune grass spreading,
the stones beneath you with their weak weak color,
the wintery seeds stayed close to other seeds
and lived on vanishing,

once they had felt the presence of the others
they didn't need anything
they couldn't add to their existence, in any way—

Empty Shadow

—In the empty city of proud joy you lay awake.
And why do you think you were called into this world,
refuser.
You whom I could not save.

You sat in the day cafes and the night cafes
and it helped to look at the lover in his beauty,
to hear delicious sentences, his sentences
had fingertips that soothed the daily wars in you,
you overheard marigolds
, by night, the chloroform bushes,
in the upstairs cafe, lowered cubes of sugar
till the upper half dissolved,
felt the oven's fury
as the firelord removed the little pizza—so solid
it would "stick to your ribs"
and you loved the food groups, the dough
went down, stick, swallow
bounce-bounce-bounce, bounce,
till it reached the sacred hollowness in you . . .

No really.
Why do you think you were called into this world.
Did you, have to, did you
have to be a something every single minute?

In the morning the mailman steps lightly over his shadow,
his mace can going tinny clink-clink
against the keys. The Friday doctor drives by
telling stories to his carphone, whole
Italies of them, and he feels special,

the fallen angel flutters down
past the eye on the dollar bill,
through the rings of Saturn and the spiral world,
he wanted God to love him but God didn't

so he keeps falling,
if I'm not loved I will keep falling,
if I'm not loved I'm empty nothing (nothing)

and your job was always to be there
when he landed, helpless in his fury,
remember lying on the cool ground in grade school,
the seed and the crumbled moments filling you in,
that wasn't so bad now was it, non-non-non-non-
light, non-God, non-mommy,
non anything near;

just lie there. That's it.
You were called to be loved
when you weren't here—

Bright Existence

In spring, the great pines waited a little faster.
Wildflowers turned
on their big circles, under the earth

and the orchid, which always came back
to the same slanty light
in the forest floor
pushed toward the edges of itself.

Lovers, are you there? Why were you one body
in that moist boat. The flower
could touch you everywhere like a party,
that series of bright confetti
in its throat—

Joy! What is it. Where does it come from;
where does it go? Sunlight
seized the flat leaves;

there should be more witnesses at the edges of the self
where everything is both.

The oak moths,
holding pale tomorrows,
dropped on invisible threads before the flower,

the part that wasn't ready
stayed inside a little longer
and the part that was ready to be something
came forth—

The Snakeskin

—And the world bent into the wide,
the field of beige and mild forevers
but the snake wanted something else;

I found its skin of stretchy diamonds
and picked it up, so I could keep
one of the two selves. The skin had eyes and the eyes

had skin, all papery before and afterward,
a little cellophane with dirt
around the rim—that's good;

there had been time for it to be one thing
before the world behind the world
called the snake, and the snake went—

UNIVERSITY PRESS OF NEW ENGLAND publishes books under its own imprint and is the publisher for Brandeis University Press, Brown University Press, University of Connecticut, Dartmouth College, Middlebury College Press, University of New Hampshire, University of Rhode Island, Tufts University, University of Vermont, and Wesleyan University Press.

ABOUT THE AUTHOR

Brenda Hillman won two awards for her first book of poetry, *White Dress,* a Wesleyan New Poets book published in 1985, the Delmore Schwartz Memorial Award from New York University and the Norma Farber First Book Award from the Poetry Society of America. She received an NEA fellowship to work on *Fortress,* her second book (1989), and received a Silver Medal from the Commonwealth Club for it. Her third book, *Death Tractates,* was published in 1992. She teaches writing at St. Mary's College, Moraga, California, and lives in Kensington, on a hill overlooking Berkeley. Hillman is a graduate of Pomona College (B.A. 1973) and of the University of Iowa (M.F.A. 1976).

LIBRARY OF CONGRESS CATALOGING-IN-PUBLICATION DATA
Hillman, Brenda.
    Bright existence / Brenda Hillman.
        p.   cm. — (Wesleyan poetry)
    Includes bibliographical references.
    ISBN 0–8195–2204–X. — ISBN 0–8195–1207–9 (pbk.)
    I. Title.   II. Series.
PS3558.I4526B75   1993
811'.54—dc20   92–53862